AN
ASPIRIN
A DAY

Also by Michael Castleman

*Before You Call the Doctor: The Family
Physician's Self-Care Guide* (with Anne
Simons, M.D., and Bobbie Hasselbring)
*The Healing Herbs: The Ultimate Guide to the
Curative Powers of Nature's Medicines*
*Sexual Solutions: For Men and the Women Who
Love Them*
*Crime-Free: The Community Crime Prevention
Handbook*
*Cold Cures: The Complete Guide to Preventing
and Treating the Common Cold and Flu*
The Medical Self-Care Book of Women's Health
(with Sadja Greenwood, M.D., and Bobbie
Hasselbring)

AN
ASPIRIN
A DAY

WHAT YOU CAN DO TO PREVENT HEART ATTACK, STROKE, AND CANCER

MICHAEL CASTLEMAN

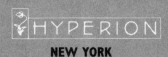

NEW YORK

Library of Congress Cataloging-in-Publication Data

Castleman, Michael.
An aspirin a day : what you can do to prevent heart attack, stroke, and cancer / by Michael Castleman. — 1st ed.
p. cm.
Includes bibliographical references and index.
ISBN 1-56282-880-0
1. Aspirin. 2. Coronary heart disease—Prevention. 3. Cerebrovascular disease—Prevention. 4. Cancer—Prevention.
I. Title.
RM666.A82C37 1993
615'.783—dc20   92-36368
CIP

10 9 8 7 6 5 4 3 2

Note: *An Aspirin a Day* is intended to familiarize readers with the latest research about this remarkable drug. However, individual differences often play an important role in medical decision-making, and neither aspirin nor the information in this book substitutes for appropriate medical care. For concerns about your specific medical situation, including the advisability of taking aspirin regularly, consult your physician.

For Maya Simons Castleman

Acknowledgments

Thanks to Martha Kaplan and Victoria DiStasio at Hyperion; Katinka Matson and John Brockman at John Brockman and Associates; Janice Guthrie and Julie Smith at The Health Resource, Conway, Arkansas; Charles C. Mann and Mark L. Plummer, coauthors of *The Aspirin Wars* (Knopf, 1991); Daniel Schuster, M.D.; the University of California's San Francisco Medical Center Library; The Aspirin Foundation, Washington, D.C.; and my family: Anne Simons, M.D., and Jeffrey and Maya Castleman.

—MICHAEL CASTLEMAN

"If aspirin were only half as effective, but cost ten times as much and were available only by prescription, maybe doctors would recommend it more frequently to prevent and treat heart attack."

—*CHARLES HENNEKENS,*
Harvard Medical School and
coauthor of Physicians' Health Study

"When it comes to medical advice, I take everything my doctor says with a grain of aspirin."

—*HENNY YOUNGMAN*

Contents

Preface

Aspirin may have saved my life. Always in good health, I thought—reasonably—that my chances of having a heart attack were small. Then last year, at age 42, I began suffering dull but severe chest pain while playing racquetball. As a physician, I knew that a heart attack was a definite possibility. Tests at an emergency room quickly confirmed it.

But as luck would have it, I had taken two aspirin several hours earlier because of a sore throat. The tests showed that the blood clot which had formed in one of my coronary arteries began to dissolve on its own almost immediately. As a result, what might have been a fatal heart attack turned out to be a mild one, leaving me with remarkably little heart damage. Sometimes the blood clots that trigger heart attacks dissolve by themselves. But aspirin makes this much more likely. That's why I believe those two little white pills may have saved my life.

There's a lot more to aspirin than relieving headaches. In *An Aspirin a Day,* you'll learn about the many amazing new uses for this familiar drug—prevention of heart attack, stroke, and other conditions. *An Aspirin a Day* is informative, comprehensive, thoroughly researched, and well written. It does an excellent job translating the technical research literature into popular terms.

The public needs to know more about aspirin's astonishing value in preventive medicine. Millions of Americans who might benefit from aspirin are not taking it. If you have any risk factors for heart attack or stroke—particularly a family his-

tory; high blood pressure; smoking; or elevated cholesterol—
I'd urge you to read *An Aspirin a Day*. Then ask your physician if you should take low-dose aspirin regularly. Some-
day, it just might save your life.

—DANIEL SCHUSTER, M.D.,
DIRECTOR,
Medical Intensive Care Unit,
Barnes Hospital,
St. Louis, Missouri, and
Associate Professor of Medicine,
Washington University School
of Medicine

AN
ASPIRIN
A DAY

THE WONDER DRUG THAT WORKS *MIRACLES*

Bayer calls its aspirin "The Wonder Drug That Works Wonders." The problem with this widely advertised phrase—one that ranks as a mortal sin for advertising copy writers—is that it *undersells* the product. Bayer's slogan ought to be "The Wonder Drug That Works *Miracles*."

Of course, "miracles" is a strong word, but after you've read *An Aspirin a Day,* chances are you'll agree it's justified. For several years now, leading researchers in cardiovascular medicine, which deals with heart disease, stroke, and related conditions, have been calling aspirin "the greatest preventive medical bargain of all time." More recently, physicians in other specialties have jumped on the aspirin bandwagon. Based on the latest research, here's just some of what this miraculous medicine now appears to do:

Aspirin reduces heart attack risk 30 to 40 percent. About 1.5 million Americans suffer heart attacks a year. Heart attack is the nation's leading cause of death, killing approximately 500,000 Americans annually. Studies to date show that regular aspirin use might prevent as many as 600,000 heart attacks a year and 200,000 heart attack deaths. (In this context, "prevent" does not mean eliminate forever but rather "postpone." Everyone eventually dies of something. Some people helped by aspirin still suffer heart attacks—and die from them—years later, or they die of something else. But aspirin helps prevents *premature* heart attacks and heart attack deaths. In other words, it helps people live longer.)

Aspirin reduces stroke risk 18 percent. Stroke is the nation's third leading killer. Aspirin helps prevent one of the two major types, ischemic stroke (explained in Chapter 2), which strikes an estimated 400,000 Americans each year, killing about 100,000 and seriously disabling tens of thousands more. If current estimates are accurate, regular aspirin use could help prevent 72,000 strokes a year, and more than 25,000 stroke-related deaths and disabilities.

Aspirin may reduce colon cancer deaths by up to 40 percent. Cancer of the colon and rectum (colorectal cancer) strikes 156,000 Americans each year and kills 60,000. It's the nation's second leading cause of cancer death (after lung cancer), and the leading cause of cancer death among nonsmokers. If current estimates are correct, regular aspirin use might prevent 24,000 colorectal cancer deaths annually.

In addition, aspirin may help prevent several other life-threatening conditions, not to mention its traditional uses for treatment of fever, pain, and inflammation.

These startling assertions are based on more than 1,000 studies published in dozens of leading medical journals over the last thirty years—about two hundred of which are listed in the References at the back of this book. But for argument's sake, let's suppose that these studies overrate aspirin's bene-fits. Let's suppose it's only *half* as beneficial as current stud-ies suggest. In that case, aspirin would prevent "only" 300,000 heart attacks, 36,000 strokes, and 12,000 colorectal cancer deaths each year. Those figures still represent a tremendous benefit. In addition, the aspirin dose physicians recommend to prevent these and other serious conditions is low, safe for most people, and costs less than a penny a day. No wonder leading researchers call aspirin "miraculous."

Physicians now urge hundreds of thousands of Americans to take an aspirin a day (or half an aspirin, or one low-strength aspirin—see Chapter 11). More and more doctors take low-dose aspirin regularly themselves.

But despite extensive news coverage—including cover sto-ries in the leading newsmagazines—most Americans remain in the dark about aspirin's amazing preventive medical value, and still consider the familiar white pills little more than an old stand-by for headaches. It's time the general public learned why aspirin has generated so much scientific excitement. *An Aspirin a Day* summarizes aspirin research through mid-1992 and discusses many benefits even your doctor may not know.

Of course, aspirin is no cure-all for heart disease, stroke, colorectal cancer, or the other conditions discussed here. No drug is. Regular aspirin use is *no substitute* for a proper diet, exercise, weight loss, stress management, smoking cessation, and medical care, particularly for those at risk for any of the conditions it helps prevent. But if physicians were ever jus-tified in telling adults, "Take two aspirins and call me in the morning," now they're equally justified in saying, "Take one aspirin a day and you may not have to call me at all."

SHOULD *YOU* TAKE ASPIRIN REGULARLY?

Quite possibly. But don't run to your medicine cabinet just yet. Be sure to read Chapters 8 and 9, which deal with aspi-

rin's side effects, interactions, the conditions it may aggravate, and how aspirin stacks up against its over-the-counter
competitors. Then you'll be ready to consider Chapter 11,
which explores two issues most physicians still consider controversial: Who should take aspirin regularly? And how much
should they take? Of course, when in doubt about the advisability of taking any drug, including aspirin, consult your
physician.

A NOTE ABOUT MEDICAL TERMINOLOGY

An Aspirin a Day holds medical jargon to a minimum. But a
few dozen technical terms have been included to familiarize
readers with the words their physicians are likely to use when
discussing the advisability of regular aspirin use. Medical terms
are explained in the text as they occur.

A NOTE ABOUT THE MEDICAL REFERENCES

All the studies cited are listed in the References at the back
of the book. If you'd like to examine any in more detail,
medical journals can be obtained at any medical school library, or at many hospital libraries. If you don't have easy
access to a medical library, ask at your public library. Many
now have computer systems capable of retrieving summaries
of journal articles using the MEDLINE database. If your local
library can't help, contact The Health Resource, a medical
research service that provides personalized computer searches
of the medical literature for a modest fee, at 209 Katherine
Drive, Conway, AR 72032; (501) 329-5272. Planetree Health
Resource Center, a consumer medical library, also offers cus-
tom searchers of the medical literature. Contact Planetree at
2040 Webster Street, San Francisco, CA 94115; (415) 923-
3680.

CHAPTER ONE

ASPIRIN HELPS PREVENT AND TREAT HEART ATTACK AND ANGINA

For almost a century, aspirin has been the world's most widely used drug for fever, aches and pains, arthritis, and other inflammatory conditions. Each year, Americans spend more than $1 billion on aspirin products, swallowing about 30 billion pills containing the drug. That's 20 tons of aspirin annually—or the equivalent of 10 tablets per person per month. Even by conservative estimates, in the future, aspirin consumption should soar as our aging population suffers more aches, pains, and arthritis—and as news of aspirin's remarkable preventive value spreads.

Aspirin has been an official medical miracle only since the late 1980s, when the Physicians' Health Study, discussed later in this chapter, confirmed its value in heart attack prevention. But the aspirin–heart attack story actually goes back more than forty years to an almost forgotten ear, nose, and throat specialist named Lawrence L. Craven, who practiced in what was then the little Los Angeles suburb of Glendale. Craven first suggested that aspirin might help prevent heart attack shortly after World War II.

Craven was raised in Iowa, received his M.D. from the University of Minnesota, and spent his professional life in Southern California. After World War II, as baby boom children began developing tonsillitis, Craven was quick to remove the infected throat glands. Tonsillectomy is rarely performed today, but in the late 1940s, it was quite common. Starting in 1948, in an effort to relieve his young patients' postsurgical throat pain, Craven prescribed a daily regimen of four sticks of Aspergum, a chewable form of aspirin.

After a tonsillectomy, incisional bleeding (hemorrhage) is possible. Not many of Craven's patients bled significantly, but some did, a few so badly that they had to be hospitalized. Most physicians would have accepted these occasional hospitalizations as unfortunate, but unremarkable, manifestations of individual differences. But Craven was unusually curious. He quizzed the hospitalized children and their parents. "In every instance of severe hemorrhage," he wrote in a 1950 letter to the *Annals of Western Medicine and Surgery,* a small professional journal, "the patient had not only chewed the four sticks of Aspergum per day, but had purchased an additional supply, consuming up to 20 sticks a day." Twenty sticks of Aspergum provides the equivalent dose of more than a dozen standard aspirin tablets.

Aspirin's connection to bleeding was nothing new. The drug, chemically known as acetylsalicylic acid, had been known to prolong bleeding and impede clotting since its nineteenth-century precursor, salicylic acid, was used to treat arthritis. Craven took the aspirin-anticlotting observation a crucial step further. He wondered if aspirin might help prevent the *internal* blood clots (thrombi) whose formation in the coronary arteries cut off the blood supply to parts of the heart and trigger heart attack. (To physicians, "clots" form only on the skin surface. Internal "clots" are called "thrombi," singular "thrombus.")

At the time, physicians were beginning to prescribe another anticoagulant, dicumarol, to men who'd had heart attacks (medically known as myocardial infarctions or MIs, literally "death of the heart wall"). In his *Annals* letter, Craven speculated that aspirin might be just as effective but cheaper and safer. (Dicumarol, it turned out, is little more than aspirin. In the blood it becomes aspirinlike salicylic acid.)

Heart disease researchers greeted Craven's 1950 article with thundering silence. And no wonder. It was published in a regional general-practice journal few heart disease researchers read. It concerned not some newly synthesized compound that might become a medical breakthrough but a drug so familiar that it was the stuff of clichés—"Take two and call me . . ." In addition, Craven wasn't in the club. The world of medical research is snobby. Full-time scientists with university affiliations have always looked down on "hobbyist" researchers with practices in the suburbs. Finally, Craven's conclusions were highly speculative. He conducted no experiment and had no statistically significant results. All he had was a crazy idea based on extrapolations from limited, potentially biased, personal observations of children. No wonder he was ignored.

Undaunted, Craven began recommending one standard 325 milligram (mg) aspirin tablet a day to men he knew who'd had heart attacks and to men who were overweight or led sedentary lives, the major risk factors known at that time. By 1953, he'd enrolled 1,465 men age 45 to 65 in his human study, or clinical trial. (*Note:* In the United States, a standard aspirin tablet contains 325 mg of the drug. In England, the standard is 5 grains. A grain is a medieval measure based on the weight of an average grain of wheat, later set at 64.8 mg. Five grains comes to 324 mg. Some aspirin studies discussed in this book have used the British 324 mg standard. Others have used the American standard of 325. The 1 mg difference has no clinical significance. For all practical purposes, the two dosages are identical.)

"It is common knowledge," Craven wrote in a report that year in an even more obscure professional publication, the *Mississippi Valley Medical Journal,* "that [overweight men who get little exercise] are more frequently and earlier in their lives exposed to the dangers of sudden coronary thrombosis"—that is, a blood clot in a coronary artery, a heart attack. In his 1953 report, he claimed that none of the men he'd put on aspirin had suffered either heart attack or unstable angina (severe chest pain while at rest, often a precursor of heart attack). "In such a large number of subjects of the type most likely to experience coronary episodes it is, to say the least, remarkable that all have remained healthy and active. This finding is contrary to statistical expectations, as well as to the experience of 36 years in practice." Craven was well aware that his clinical trial was not methodologically rigorous, and he invited full-time researchers to pursue his lead. No one did.

Meanwhile, Craven continued his trial, and in his final report, a 1956 article in the *Mississippi Valley Medical Journal,* he claimed 8,000 enrollees and truly astonishing results: no detectable heart attacks, and no detectable strokes. Nine of his 8,000 subjects had died of suspected heart attacks, but on autopsy, their deaths were attributed to burst arteries (aneurysms), not to coronary thrombi. "Surely," Craven wrote, "[taking one aspirin a day] could do no harm. . . . It might even prove lifesaving. . . . Aspirin administration offers a safe and sure method of [preventing] coronary thrombosis."

Craven was right, but his research methods left much to be desired. He never made sure that his 8,000 subjects actually took an aspirin a day. He did not control the other drugs they took, which could easily have confounded his results. He had no control group who took a placebo for comparison purposes. And he already believed in the effectiveness of the treatment he was prescribing, which raised the specter of experimental bias. (Today, critics think Craven might even have fudged his data. They say that despite aspirin, in any group of 8,000 middle-aged men followed for six years, *someone* should have had a heart attack.)

As astonishing as his 1956 claims were, heart disease researchers continued to ignore Craven. And had anyone been interested, his death the following year would surely have given them pause. The seventy-four-year-old daily aspirin taker dropped dead suddenly—of a heart attack.

Today, more than thirty years after Craven's death, heart disease authorities consider his work prophetic. As James E. Dalen, M.D., editor of *Archives of Internal Medicine,* wrote in 1991, "One can only wonder what the impact of Craven's recommendations might have been if they had appeared in a medical publication with a wider circulation than the *Mississippi Valley Medical Journal.* If Craven's 'aspirin a day' rule had been adopted in 1950, hundreds of thousands of myocardial infarctions and strokes might have been prevented."

THE NATION'S LEADING KILLER

The heart and blood vessels form the cardiovascular system ("cardio" means "heart"; "vascular" refers to the blood vessels). Cardiovascular diseases—primarily heart disease and stroke—are by far the nation's leading causes of death. Of the nation's 2.2 million deaths each year, cardiovascular diseases account for 900,000 (42 percent), or one death every 34 seconds. Of that total, heart diseases claim 765,000 lives (35 percent of U.S. deaths), and strokes kill 150,500 (7 percent). Cardiovascular diseases are *twice* as lethal as cancer, which claims 485,000 lives a year (22 percent of the nation's deaths).

Among the many heart diseases, two major ones are heart

attack and angina. Each year, 1.5 million Americans suffer heart attacks and about 500,000 die from them. The nation's death rate from heart attack has plummeted about 40 percent since 1960, but myocardial infarction still ranks as the nation's leading killer. Meanwhile, 6 million Americans have angina, which places them at high risk for heart attack.

Both heart attack and angina are "coronary artery diseases." The coronary arteries circle the heart and provide food and oxygen to the remarkable muscle that beats *3 billion* times during the average lifetime. ("Coronary" comes from the Latin *corona* meaning "encircling.") Coronary artery disease develops when these major blood vessels become narrowed (occluded) by cholesterol-rich deposits that build up on their inner walls. The clogging process is called "atherosclerosis." (In Greek, *athero* means "paste," and *sklerosis* means "thickening.") The deposits are known as atherosclerotic plaques. An estimated 70 percent of the U.S. population has coronary artery disease to some extent. It often begins in childhood.

Scientists are uncertain precisely how atherosclerosis occurs, but the leading theory is that chemical changes in the blood caused by smoking; a high-fat, high-cholesterol diet; and the other risk factors for heart disease soon to be discussed more fully injure the artery lining. The injuries attract the body's first line of defense against bleeding, special blood cells called "platelets," which clump together at the injury site. Over time, the platelets are joined by fats, cholesterol, calcium, cellular debris, and other clotting factors, forming a plaque.

Sometimes, when atherosclerosis significantly diminishes blood flow to the heart, the result is stable angina—severe chest pain during physical activity that subsides with rest. In more serious cases, chest pain occurs even while resting (unstable angina). Angina itself is not fatal, but those who suffer it are at high risk for heart attack.

A heart attack occurs when an atherosclerotic plaque ruptures, rather like a pimple popping. The rupture triggers the formation of a thrombus. If the thrombus lodges inside an already severely narrowed coronary artery, it blocks blood flow, causing serious damage to part of the heart, and the often crushing chest pain of a heart attack.

Heart attack chest pain usually lasts thirty minutes or longer and often radiates up to the jaw or down an arm. Other heart attack symptoms include sweating, nausea, vomiting, dizziness, and fainting. Some people say they experience premonitions of doom beforehand. (Not all heart attacks cause severe chest pain. Some feel like heartburn. See page 40.)

A heart attack can come on gradually, preceded by a few weeks of angina, or strike without warning. About one-third of those who have heart attacks don't survive them. Most deaths occur within two hours, often before the victim reaches an emergency medical facility.

Coronary artery disease does not strike suddenly. It's the culmination of a process that takes decades. The odds of developing this modern plague depend on several risk factors. Some can be voluntarily controlled; others cannot. Risk factors that cannot be changed include:

Heredity. If heart disease runs in your family, you're at increased risk. You're not necessarily *fated* to develop coronary artery disease, but you've probably inherited a tendency toward atherosclerosis. In addition, several other coronary artery disease risk factors have genetic components: diabetes, obesity, high blood pressure (hypertension), and elevated cholesterol levels (familial hypercholesterolemia).

Gender. Men suffer more heart attacks than women, and they occur earlier in life. Few women have heart attacks in their 40s or early 50s. Compared with men, however, women over 65 are more than twice as likely to die within a few weeks of a heart attack.

Increasing age. More than half of all heart attacks strike people over 65. Of those people killed by them, about 80 percent are over 65.

Diabetes. Cardiovascular diseases claim the lives of more than 80 percent of diabetics. An estimated 12 million Americans have diabetes, which occurs when the body stops producing the pancreatic hormone insulin, or becomes unable to use the insulin it produces. Without insulin, the cells cannot consume blood sugar (glucose), the body's major fuel. There are two kinds of diabetes: Type 1, where diabetics must inject insulin, and Type 2, which can usually be controlled through weight loss and diet. Type 2 is far more prevalent, accounting for 85 to 90 percent of cases. Diabetes is a serious chronic disease that requires ongoing professional care. In addition to cardiovascular disease, diabetes may also cause blindness and serious kidney and nerve damage.

Prior heart attack or angina. Most people with a history of heart attack or angina have significant coronary artery disease—and a substantially increased risk of a subsequent heart attack.

Risk factors for coronary artery disease that can be changed include:

Smoking. Smokers' risk of heart attack is twice that of nonsmokers, and smokers who have heart attacks are more likely to die from them. Smoking damages the blood vessels, makes the platelets stickier, and accelerates development of atherosclerosis. The nicotine in cigarette smoke raises blood pressure, and the carbon monoxide reduces the amount of oxygen the blood can carry. Smoking is also the main risk factor for peripheral vascular disease, atherosclerotic narrowing of the arteries that carry blood to the arms and legs. When this condition becomes severe, the treatment is amputation.

High blood pressure. As atherosclerosis narrows the arteries, the heart must work harder to pump blood through them. This extra effort makes the blood push harder against the artery walls, raising blood pressure. Hypertension is called the "silent killer" because for years it causes no symptoms. But over time, as the heart becomes chronically overworked, it can become seriously weakened. Hypertension also increases risk of stroke and kidney failure.

Blood pressure is measured by two numbers. The first, systolic pressure, measures the force in the arteries during heartbeats, when the heart is pumping. The second, diastolic, measures the residual pressure between heartbeats, when the heart is resting. Textbook normal blood pressure in an adult is 120/80, but this figure is misleading. Normal blood pressure actually ranges up to 140/90. Above that level, it's high.

Physicians view normal blood pressure as a range because it fluctuates considerably during the day. It's lower in the morning, higher in the afternoon and evening. It also rises with stressful events and some drugs, and with increasing age as the arteries lose some of their flexibility. If you feel tense during a doctor visit, you may even develop a temporary blood pressure increase (white coat hypertension).

High cholesterol. Cholesterol is a fatlike substance found in every cell in the human body. It's necessary for healthy cell membranes and other vital functions. The problem with cholesterol is that many people have too much in their blood. Blood (serum) cholesterol comes from two sources: synthesis in the liver, and certain foods in the diet, especially high-fat animal products—eggs, red meats, and whole-milk dairy products. The liver makes all the cholesterol the body needs. The cholesterol associated with coronary artery disease comes from the diet.

Serum cholesterol is measured by the amount (in milligrams, or mg) found in a certain volume of blood (deciliter, or dl). Experts disagree on the level considered heart-safe.

Heart attack is extremely rare among people whose total cholesterol is 150 mg/dl or less. Risk increases as cholesterol level rises, and risk accelerates sharply at levels above 200 mg/dl, which is why the American Heart Association urges everyone to keep their cholesterol below 200. Unfortunately, about half of adult Americans have cholesterol levels above 200, and among men over 45 and women over 60, the age groups at greatest risk for heart attack, more than one-third have cholesterol levels above 240.

Cholesterol tests typically measure total cholesterol, but those with levels above 200 may have their reading divided into LDL, or low-density lipoproteins, and HDL, high-density lipoproteins. Lipoproteins are special molecules that carry cholesterol in the blood. LDL molecules carry about two-thirds of circulating cholesterol, and LDL cholesterol is most closely associated with the growth of atherosclerotic plaques. The higher the LDL level, the greater the risk of coronary artery disease. That's why LDL is called "bad cholesterol." LDL should be no higher than 130 mg/dl.

HDL, on the other hand, is "good." It clears circulating cholesterol out of the bloodstream. The higher the HDL reading, the *lower* the risk of coronary artery disease. HDL should be no lower than 40 mg/dl.

Obesity. Even with no other risk factors for coronary artery disease, people who are obese—the medical term for weighing at least 20 percent more than the recommended figure for their height and build—are at increased risk for heart attack and stroke. Obesity is strongly associated with high blood pressure because the heart must work harder to pump blood through so much extra tissue. Obesity is also associated with elevated cholesterol levels and lack of exercise.

Recent research shows that *where* people carry their extra weight is almost as important as how much extra weight they carry. A fat stomach ("apple shape" or "beer belly") is more hazardous than fat hips ("pear shape" or "saddle bags").

Sedentary life-style. The heart is a muscle, and the rule that applies to other muscles applies equally to the heart: Use it or lose it. Regular moderate exercise helps condition the heart. A sedentary life-style deconditions it. A sedentary life-style is also associated with other heart attack risk factors: smoking, obesity, and elevated cholesterol and blood pressure.

Type-A behavior. "Type-A" refers to a particular group of stress-related traits: impatience, hostility, and feeling constantly time-pressured. Type-A's don't walk; they run. They are forever trying to squeeze more accomplishments into less time. They interrupt others. They yell at other drivers. They don't have the time or patience for much socializing. They hate to wait for anything, and they especially resent lines in supermarkets and at toll booths. When friends and loved ones urge them to slow down and lighten up, they dismiss the idea as impossible or ridiculous. The Framingham Heart Study, the nation's oldest and largest ongoing investigation of heart disease risk factors, has shown that Type-A behavior doubles the risk of heart attack in men over 50 and triples it in women.

Birth control pills. Oral contraceptives increase the likelihood of thrombus formation (thrombosis). As a result, Pill use contributes to the risk of many cardiovascular diseases: heart attack, stroke, pulmonary embolism (an arterial obstruction in one of the lungs), and thrombophlebitis (thrombus formation in the major veins, often in the legs). Risk is greatest for Pill users over 35 who smoke or have a personal or family history of cardiovascular disease, diabetes, hypertension, or elevated cholesterol.

THOSE PESKY PLATELETS

A century ago, the leading causes of death in the United States were all infectious diseases such as tuberculosis. Heart attacks were extremely rare, in part because few people lived into their sixties, the period when myocardial infarction becomes most prevalent today, and in part because heart attack risk factors were less of a problem—people smoked less, got more exercise, ate a diet lower in fat, and were less likely to be obese or Type-A. In fact, physicians didn't pay much attention to heart attack until after World War I, when heart attack deaths started to rise just as antibiotics and such public health measures as modern sewage systems began to control the infectious diseases. By 1940, heart attack was the nation's leading cause of death, and by the mid-1950s, when Craven conducted his aspirin studies, it had become a plague.

Columbia University researcher Harvey J. Weiss had never heard of Craven, but a decade after the California physician's death, Weiss unwittingly followed in his footsteps with a modest article in the prestigious British medical journal *The Lancet*. Weiss's paper answered a seventy-year-old medical mystery—why aspirin prolongs bleeding. Weiss showed that the drug chemically interferes with clotting.

Platelets, named because early anatomists thought they looked like tiny plates, are disklike cells about one-third the size of oxygen-carrying red blood cells. Made by the bone marrow, platelets are incredibly numerous—200,000 to 300,000 per cubic milliliter of blood, with billions in the total blood supply.

Weiss believed that when blood vessels become injured, circulating platelets attracted to the wound released a substance called "adenosine diphosphate" (ADP), which increased platelet stickiness, causing the tiny cells to clump together at the injury site. Known as platelet aggregation, this, in turn, attracted other blood elements involved in injury repair, and eventually a clot or thrombus formed that resealed the damaged blood vessel and prevented continued bleeding.

Weiss discovered that aspirin interferes with the platelets' release of ADP, thus slowing platelet aggregation and prolonging bleeding. He and coauthor Louis M. Aledort, of New York's Albert Einstein School of Medicine, suggested that aspirin "might have antitithrombotic properties," meaning that it might prevent arterial thrombi. Other researchers confirmed the Weiss-Aledort findings and suggested that aspirin might help prevent the two most catastrophic thrombotic events—heart attack and ischemic stroke, which occurs when a thrombus stops blood flow to part of the brain. (The other major type of stroke is caused by bleeding inside the brain, hemmorhagic stroke—see Chapter 2.)

Speculation about aspirin's possible antithrombotic value piqued immediate interest among rheumatologists (physicians who specialize in treating arthritis). For years, rheumatologists had been puzzled by a curious observation: Heart attacks seemed to strike a surprisingly small fraction of elderly rheumatoid arthritis sufferers. Rheumatoid arthritis (RA) is among the most serious forms of the painful joint disease, and those who have it often take a great deal of aspirin— 4,000 to 8,000 mg (12 to 25 standard tablets) a day. Might RA sufferers' aspirin consumption explain their unexpected freedom from MI?

To answer this question, in 1974 University of California researchers compared the autopsy records of 62 elderly RA sufferers with those of 62 similar people (matched controls) whose medical histories suggested that they were not regular users of aspirin. The coronary arteries of both groups showed similar evidence of atherosclerosis. If aspirin prevented heart attack, it did not do it by preventing the growth of plaques. But the RA group showed only one-third as many heart attacks—7 compared with 21 in the control group—a highly

significant difference. The only difference the researchers could
find was the arthritis sufferers' steady consumption of aspirin.

The researchers also examined aspirin's effect on stroke.
If aspirin prevented coronary thrombosis, it should do the
same in the brain, and reduce the risk of arterial blockages
and ischemic stroke. Indeed, the RA group showed fewer
ischemic strokes—10 versus 14 in the control group—but the
difference was not statistically significant. It could have happened by chance.

On the other hand, since aspirin prolongs bleeding, one
might suspect that regular aspirin use would increase risk of
hemorrhagic stroke. But the RA sufferers experienced significantly fewer hemorrhagic strokes—only two versus seven in
the control group. These results were quite exciting. Aspirin
appeared to reduce risk of heart attack and possibly ischemic
stroke without increasing risk of hemorrhagic stroke.

Off the record, the researchers probably batted about the
term *miracle,* but on the record they remained cautious. Their
study had been "retrospective." They'd started with certain
facts—autopsy findings—and looked back in time to see if
they could find any differences in behavior—regular versus
occasional aspirin use. "In spite of the obvious attractions of
the aspirin hypothesis," they wrote in the journal *Arthritis
and Rheumatism,* "the data do not permit the conclusion that
aspirin prevented heart attacks in the patients with rheumatoid arthritis. Only prospective controlled studies can determine this."

By "prospective," they meant following a large group of
subjects over time as Craven had. By "controlled," they meant
using state-of-the-art methodology: a placebo-controlled, randomized, double-blind design.

• "Placebo-controlled" meant giving half the subjects aspirin and the other half a lookalike but chemically inert placebo.

- "Randomized" meant assigning subjects to the aspirin and placebo groups at random.
- And "double-blind" meant that neither the subjects nor the researchers could know who got what. This keeps the placebo subjects from sabotaging the study by taking aspirin, and the researchers from allowing their biases to cloud the results.

Unfortunately, prospective, placebo-controlled, randomized, double-blind clinical trials are very expensive. To produce valid results, they must follow large numbers of subjects for several years. Of course, the more subjects and the longer the follow-up, the higher the cost, so researchers often wind up walking a fine line between scientific validity and financial feasibility.

SEVEN FATEFUL CLINICAL TRIALS

Despite the high cost of large, scientifically rigorous clinical trials, the possibility that cheap, convenient, reasonably safe aspirin might help prevent the nation's first and third leading causes of death was certainly worth investigating, and from 1971 to 1983, the results of seven clinical trials were published.

The first, by Finnish researchers, was a complete bust. For one year, they gave 430 people over age 70 a daily dose of either a placebo or 1,000 mg of aspirin (about three standard tablets). Their results showed no differences whatsoever in death or hospitalization rates for heart attack or stroke. On the other hand, aspirin did not increase risk of hemorrhagic stroke. Writing in the *Journal of the American Geriatrics Society,* the researchers were clearly disappointed. They'd gone to a good deal of trouble to test a promising treatment and had come up with nothing. Today, researchers believe that this study's subjects were simply too old. Aspirin works its MI- and stroke-preventive magic best in people under 70. When this study was published in 1971, however, its results weighed heavily against aspirin. Aspirin's clinical trial score read: zero studies pro, one solidly con.

The second trial, a British study, was published in 1974 by Peter C. Elwood, M.D., of the Medical Research Council Epidemiology Unit in Cardiff, South Wales. It examined aspirin use and the risk of second heart attacks in men who'd already had one. For one year, the researchers put 1,239 male heart attack survivors on a daily regimen of either a placebo or 300 mg of aspirin (slightly less than one standard tablet). After six months the aspirin group showed 12 percent fewer deaths from second heart attacks, and after a year 25 percent fewer deaths. Unfortunately, the reductions were not statistically significant; they could have occurred by chance. Writing in the *British Medical Journal,* Elwood had to dismiss his results as "inconclusive," making the score: one study insignificantly pro, one solidly con.

Elwood's 25 percent reduction in heart attack deaths *sounds* significant. Why wasn't it? The reason was that the subjects' death rates changed only a little. If, say, 4 percent of the controls died, and 3 percent of the aspirin users died, that would be a reduction of 25 percent, but actually only a slight change, and in a relatively small study population of 1,239, one that was not statistically significant.

At this point clinical trial authorities started wondering about Type II errors. In research, it's easy to make mistakes. Sometimes studies "find" something that turns out not to be true. This is a Type I error, which occurred, for example, in the study some years ago that linked moderate coffee consumption to an increased risk of pancreatic cancer. Subsequent studies could not replicate this finding, and after a while it was dismissed as a Type I error. On the other hand, sometimes studies fail to find something that *is* true. This is a Type II error, such as occurred in several of the early studies of vitamin C for use in treating the common cold. It turned out that these experiments used doses that were too low for too brief a period. More recently, using a higher dose (2,000 mg a day) for a longer period, three rigorous studies at the Respiratory Viruses Research Laboratory at the University of Wisconsin in Madison have shown the vitamin to have significant value in cold prevention and treatment.

Heart disease researchers felt frustrated. Aspirin's mechanism of action—its antiplatelet effect—*ought* to prevent coronary thombosis. The rheumatoid arthritis retrospective study looked great—aspirin should work. So why hadn't the first two clinical trials come up with significant benefit? Both were reasonably large, reasonably long, and well run. But perhaps they'd both made Type II errors—failed to find a real effect.

In the same issue of the *British Medical Journal* that contained Elwood's inconclusive report, another study increased suspicions of Type II errors. It was not a clinical trial, but rather a survey conducted by the Boston Collaborative Drug Surveillance Group, which compiled data from two dozen hospitals around the world. Researchers asked 776 male hospital patients who'd survived heart attacks how often they'd used aspirin, and asked the same question of 13,989 demographically similar men hospitalized for other reasons. Compared with the heart attack survivors, those who had never had heart attacks were twice as likely to have used aspirin frequently, raising the possibility that their aspirin use had helped protect them. Unfortunately, drug-recollection studies are not persuasive, because people's memories are often inaccurate. Nonetheless, the researchers concluded that their results were "consistent with the hypothesis that [regular aspirin use] confers some protection [against heart attack]."

Here was another pro-aspirin report. Everything looked *so good* for aspirin, except the most important data, the clinical trial results. As they reviewed the two disappointing trials, researchers focused on their numbers—1,239 and 776 subjects. They *seemed* large enough, but suppose they weren't?

The results might then show no significant benefit because, in fact, aspirin's real benefit had been obscured by study populations too small to show it. What was needed, the researchers decided, was a *really big* trial, something huge, even if it cost a fortune.

This argument eventually fell on receptive ears at the U.S. National Heart Lung and Blood Institute (NHLBI), a division of the National Institutes of Health. In 1975 the NHLBI launched what ranked at the time as one of the largest, most ambitious clinical trials ever attempted, the Aspirin Myocardial Infarction Study (AMIS). The three-year, $17 million experiment involved 4,200 men and women aged 30 to 69 who'd had at least one heart attack. Twice a day, half took a placebo and half took 500 mg of aspirin (the equivalent to one and a half standard tablets). AMIS was launched with great fanfare. An editorial in the *Journal of the American Medical Association* urged physicians to scour their records and encourage patients who were heart attack survivors to enroll. AMIS was so big that everyone expected it to answer the aspirin–heart attack question once and for all.

In 1976, while AMIS was gearing up, the third clinical trial was published by the Coronary Drug Research Group at the University of Maryland. Starting with 1,529 middle-aged men who'd had heart attacks, the researchers gave half a placebo, and half 324 mg of aspirin (one standard tablet). After three years, the aspirin group showed 30 percent fewer heart attack deaths. Impressive as this finding appeared, it, too, was statistically insignificant. In addition, the aspirin users complained about stomach pain twice as frequently as those in the placebo group, prompting the researchers to warn: "The availability of aspirin as a nonprescription drug, and the general belief that it poses little or no risk make [our subjects' reports of stomach pain] a potentially serious problem since aspirin is, in fact, a powerful drug that can have serious side effects." This trial made the score: two studies insignificantly pro, one solidly con.

In 1979, Peter Elwood's British group published the results of the fourth aspirin trial, which, like their earlier effort, were disappointing. This study involved 1,682 hospital patients with confirmed heart attacks (including 248 women). Upon discharge, half took a placebo three times a day; the other half took 300 mg of aspirin (slightly less than one tablet) on the same schedule. One year later, second heart attacks killed 17 percent fewer people in the aspirin group. But the difference was statistically insignificant—in fact, very insignificant. "For acceptable statistical significance," Elwood wrote in *The Lancet,* "the reductions [in heart attack among the aspirin users] would have had to have been almost double [what we found]." The score now stood: three studies insignificantly pro, one solidly con.

Then, on February 15, 1980, the *Journal of the American Medical Association* published the results of the much-anticipated AMIS study—and shattered most physicians' hopes that aspirin might prevent heart attack. Compared with the placebo group, the aspirin group's overall death rate was slightly *higher.* The aspirin users suffered 30 percent fewer nonfatal heart attacks, but like all the previous studies, the difference was not statistically significant. The observed reduction could have been a fluke. The aspirin users also suffered fewer strokes, but again, the difference was statistically insignificant. "AMIS is the largest investigation [to date] of aspirin in the post-MI population," the researchers wrote, "and more weight must be given its results. They clearly indicate that the regular administration of aspirin does not reduce three-year mortality in patients with a history of MI. Based on AMIS results, aspirin is not recommended for routine use in patients who have survived an MI."

To make matters even worse, almost twice as many aspirin takers developed ulcers and stomach inflammation, and three times as many reported stomach pain and nausea. "In the dose used (1,000 mg or about three standard tablets a day), aspirin cannot be considered innocuous."

After AMIS, the score read: four trials insignificantly pro, one solidly con. But AMIS's failure sounded the death knell for aspirin as a heart attack preventive. Despite its enormous subject pool, and $17 million cost, all AMIS had proven was that the pain reliever doctors recommend most was nothing more than that.

In the wake of the AMIS disaster, few physicians noticed the publication of the sixth aspirin trial by the German-Austrian Study Group in Frankfurt. Starting with 946 heart attack survivors—743 men and 203 women—the researchers gave half a daily placebo and half 1,500 mg of aspirin (more than four and a half standard tablets), or another anticoagulant. After seven years, the aspirin users suffered 42 percent fewer heart attack deaths than the placebo takers, and 46 percent fewer than those who took the other anticoagulant. Though impressive at first glance, the results were statistically insignificant. However, when only the men were considered, the aspirin takers suffered 56 percent fewer heart attack deaths, a difference that was significant, but just barely. Writing in the British journal *Haemostasis* ("stopping blood flow"), the European researchers concluded that male heart attack survivors "have a lower risk of coronary death if treated with 1,500 mg of ASA daily, . . . [but] ASA seems more effective in men than in women." The score, if anyone still cared, was: five studies pro (only one barely significant and only in men), and one solidly con.

Finally, in 1980, the Persantine-Aspirin Reinfarction Study Research Group weighed in the results of the seventh aspirin trial. This study involved 2,026 men and women ages 30 to 74 who'd had confirmed heart attacks. Three times a day, half took a placebo; the other half took either 324 mg of aspirin (one tablet), or aspirin plus 75 mg of Persantine (dipyridamole), another antiplatelet drug, whose manufacturer underwrote the study's $8.2 million cost. After three years of follow-up, compared with the placebo takers, the aspirin and aspirin-Persantine groups experienced approximately 20 percent fewer heart attack deaths, but again these differences were statistically insignificant.

After seven methodologically rigorous clinical trials, the final score read: six studies pro (but only one barely significant and only in men), and one solidly con. The studies showing statistically insignificant benefit had to be discarded, so the real score was: one barely pro, one solidly con. Meanwhile, the enormous AMIS study had failed to show any persuasive benefit. Researchers agreed: If AMIS couldn't show that aspirin prevents heart attack, no study could. Aspirin was dead in the water.

ASPIRIN STRIKES BACK

Three months after the AMIS results appeared, J. M. Ritter, a professor of medicine at Johns Hopkins, wrote an impassioned critique of drug-research methods that appeared in *The Lancet*. His seemingly heretical article, "Placebo-Controlled, Double-Blind Clinical Trials Can Impede Medical Progress," acknowledged the value of large subject pools, random assignment, and prospective, placebo-controlled, double-blind design; however, he argued that drug researchers had become so imprisoned by the demands of statisticians that they had developed a bad case of tunnel vision. Placebo-controlled, double-blind designs were "all well and good as far as they go," Ritter wrote, "but there is a more fundamental question: Are they sensible or not? . . . As a result of insisting on statistically impeccable [designs] we may get highly reliable answers to inherently trivial questions." Ritter then critiqued several noted studies of the day, including a 1978 Canadian report on aspirin for stroke prevention (discussed in Chapter 2). "Aspirin was not used optimally," he argued, because of a "too-slavish adherence" to an unnecessarily rigid study design. As a result, "many questions remain unanswered," among them, aspirin's role in the prevention of heart attack.

Ritter's accusation that tyrannical statisticians were destroying clinical trials struck a sensitive nerve. Unbeknownst to Ritter, many clinical trial statisticians had come to similar conclusions. They had also come up with a bold new way to answer some of his objections.

The statisticians announced their mathematical innovation later that same month, May 1980, through an editorial in *The Lancet,* which reported on the inaugural meeting of the Society for Clinical Trials in Philadelphia. Much of this high-powered conference was devoted to reanalyzing the results of the AMIS study and the five other credible aspirin–heart attack trials. (By this time, the Finnish trial with the too-elderly subjects had been discarded.)

Viewed individually, the six trials made aspirin look useless for the prevention of heart attack. *Taken as a whole,* however, as though they had all been arms of one truly enormous study, a different picture emerged, one that showed aspirin clearly beneficial for heart attack prevention. The statisticians called their new trial combination technique "meta-analysis." In effect, it enlarged subject pools, allowing small, seemingly "insignificant" differences in individual trials to add up to significant findings—if they really were significant. Meta-analysis, the statisticians insisted, proved that for prevention of heart attack, aspirin was a winner.

"In view of the arguments the [aspirin–heart attack] trials have generated," *The Lancet* editorialized, "what was surprising [about this gathering of clinical trial experts] was that a reasonably clear consensus emerged. Aspirin, it was agreed, does reduce the risk of death [from heart attack. . . . Using meta-analysis], there were [significantly] fewer deaths than expected among the aspirin patients. . . . The overall reduction in reinfarction was 21 percent."

In one fell swoop, the new Society for Clinical Trials had reestablished aspirin as a major boon to heart attack prevention. All that remained, *The Lancet* editorial continued, was to determine the optimal dose and schedule: "Doses of about 1,000 mg a day cause [gastrointestinal side effects that are] not trivial. . . . They may perhaps be reduced by the use of buffered or enteric-coated aspirin, which both seem to reduce stomach damage. [But several studies] suggest that treatment only once every two or three days with only 300 mg of aspirin may be as effective as daily treatment [with higher doses]. There are many possibilities to explore. But now we know that aspirin is worthwhile."

Given AMIS's conclusion a few short months earlier that aspirin was "not recommended" for prevention of heart attack, *The Lancet* report was extraordinary: "The pharmaceutical companies," the journal continued, "should now make aspirin available in some practical form of packaging, such as day-marked calendar packs, to help patients remember to take one tablet a day if it is so prescribed."

Sterling Drug, maker of Bayer, immediately petitioned the FDA for permission to market such an aspirin calendar pack, but the agency wouldn't hear of it. The FDA committee that denied Sterling's application was suspicious of meta-analysis. The technique was too new, too controversial. AMIS, which had been funded by the FDA's sister federal agency, had shown that aspirin was useless against heart attack. Case closed.

Over time, meta-analysis became more accepted. In 1983, Canadian researchers used the technique to reanalyze the six clinical trials, and concluded: "The combined data indicate a highly significant 21 percent reduction in reinfarction rate and a 16 percent reduction in mortality in the patients treated with aspirin." For heart attack prevention, aspirin is "most useful."

ASPIRIN REDUCES
HEART ATTACK RISK 44 PERCENT

AMIS's aftershocks were finally laid to rest in 1983, when the prestigious *New England Journal of Medicine* published the Kansas City–based Veterans Administration Cooperative Study. Using a rigorous design, the researchers enrolled 1,266 men, average age 56, with unstable angina (chest pain while at rest, which made them prime candidates for heart attack). Once a day, half took a placebo, while the other half took 324 mg of aspirin (one standard tablet). After twelve weeks, those in the aspirin group had suffered 51 percent fewer fatal and 51 percent fewer nonfatal heart attacks. Both results were highly statistically significant. In addition, the aspirin users suffered no more side effects than the placebo group. Surprisingly, aspirin's protective effect persisted long after the study ended. A year later, compared with the placebo survivors, the aspirin-group survivors experienced 43 percent fewer heart attack deaths. "This trial," the researchers concluded, "demonstrates that a single dose of 324 mg of aspirin has a highly protective effect against myocardial infarction. . . . Because of its effectiveness and safety, we recommend aspirin as a valuable addition to the management of unstable angina in men, and perhaps in women."

The Veterans study tilted the balance in aspirin's favor once and for all. The drug definitely helped prevent heart attack in those with heart disease. But what about those with no history or outward signs of heart disease? Could aspirin prevent *first* heart attacks?

Heart attack may be the nation's leading cause of death, but in the healthy population, MI's don't occur all that frequently. For a valid test of aspirin's ability to prevent first heart attacks, a prospective, randomized, double-blind, placebo-controlled study would require unbelievably huge numbers of subjects followed for many years, which meant an impossibly large price tag. AMIS had been too expensive. The federal government wouldn't hear of putting up anywhere near $17 million again.

Fortunately, two leading British epidemiologists had already come up with an elegant way to mount huge studies cheaply. One was Sir Richard Doll, who'd been knighted for his work in the 1950s proving that cigarette smoking causes lung cancer. The other was Richard Peto, a pioneer of meta-analysis. Their idea? Use physicians as subjects and follow them by mail. Doll and Peto knew that British doctors were fascinated by the aspirin–heart attack question. Their interest, they reasoned, might make them willing to participate in a trial of it themselves. They also felt confident that physicians, who appreciated the demands of research methodology, would follow directions without much supervision, allowing follow-up by mail at tremendous cost savings. Starting in 1978, they sent a letter to every male physician in the United Kingdom requesting participation in a trial of aspirin for prevention of first heart attack (primary prevention). After eliminating those who already took aspirin regularly, and those with ulcers or previous strokes or heart attack, they enrolled 5,139 subjects for their six-year British Doctors' Study. Two-thirds took 500 mg of aspirin a day; one-third was asked not to take any aspirin or other salicylates and to use acetaminophen to treat fever and pain.

Ironically, Doll and Peto knew from the outset that their subject pool was too small to produce any significant findings. But they hoped to demonstrate the feasibility of their low-rent approach so that American researchers could sell the idea to the U.S. government. If American doctors participated in a similar study, and the two sets of results were combined using meta-analysis, Doll and Peto believed the combined studies would produce significant results.

Coincidentally, Harvard epidemiologist Charles H. Hennekens happened to be spending a year in England working with Doll and Peto as they developed the British Doctors' Study. When he returned to Massachusetts, Hennekens told the National Institutes of Health (NIH) that using the Doll-Peto model, he could orchestrate a trial several times the size of AMIS for less than one-quarter of its cost, just $4 million. It took a while, but eventually NIH approved funding and the Physicians' Health Study was launched.

32   AN ASPIRIN A DAY

Hennekens's team sent a mailing to all 261,248 U.S. male physicians from age 40 to 84. Among the doctors willing to participate, they excluded those with any history of heart attack or stroke, and those who took aspirin for arthritis. By January 1984, at the start of the planned seven-year project, the Physicians' Health Study had 33,233 enrollees, of whom 22,071 finished the trial. Every other day, half the doctors took a placebo, and half took 325 mg of aspirin (one standard tablet). Both groups used the kind of calendar pill-pack *The Lancet* had suggested four years earlier.

The months passed and the data began to accumulate. Twice a year, Hennekens and a team of physicians from NIH reviewed it to see if any differences had emerged. At first, as expected, none did. All the physicians were reasonably healthy and none had had previous strokes or heart attacks, so few participants in either the aspirin or placebo groups suffered either one. But halfway through the study, a remarkable difference did turn up. The control group reported 189 heart attacks, the aspirin group only 104, a highly significant difference of more than 40 percent. The NIH steering committee decided to halt the trial immediately on the grounds that it would have been unethical to deny aspirin to the control group when taking it so clearly reduced their risk of heart attack.

On January 28, 1988, almost twenty-five years to the day after Craven originally proposed aspirin for MI prevention, the *New England Journal of Medicine* published the Physicians' Health Study's preliminary findings: Aspirin prevented first heart attacks.

Eighteen months later, the same journal published the Physicians' Health Study's final report. The NIH steering committee wrote that regular aspirin use produced "a statistically significant 44 percent reduction in risk of myocardial infarction. Our trial demonstrates conclusively a benefit of aspirin in reducing the incidence of first myocardial infarction, and thus extends the previous findings to healthy people. Since the publication of our preliminary report, 74 percent of the participants who were assigned to placebo have [started taking] aspirin.''

The results of the British Doctors' Study were published in the *British Medical Journal* just two days after the *New England Journal*'s preliminary report, but the publicity about the U.S. trial reduced the event to a footnote on this side of the Atlantic. In the British study, aspirin reduced heart attack risk 25 percent, and heart attack deaths 10 percent, but as expected the results were not statistically significant. However, when the British and U.S. doctor trials were combined, aspirin reduced risk of heart attack by about one-third.

For the record, aspirin's MI-preventive benefits emerged only in participants over age 50, but many cardiologists now recommend starting earlier for those with significant risk factors. In addition, the aspirin group suffered a small, statistically insignificant, but nonetheless disturbing, increase in hemorrhagic stroke (see Chapter 2).

Despite the concern about stroke, the combined results of the two doctor studies made regular aspirin use as important to heart attack prevention as quitting smoking, regular exercise, and cholesterol, stress, and blood pressure control. Cardiologists quickly embraced aspirin, and today it's difficult to find a heart specialist who doesn't take the drug regularly.

Other physicians have been slower to hop on the aspirin bandwagon. A 1991 survey of Canadian family physicians showed that two-thirds recommended low-dose aspirin for patients with heart disease, but that fewer than 20 percent took it themselves. And in mid-1992 in San Francisco, at an American Heart Association (AHA) seminar on cardiology for family practitioners, the cardiologist-president of the AHA's San Francisco chapter opened the meeting by asking the assembled physicians to raise their hands if they took aspirin regularly. Only a few hands went up. The speaker was incredulous: ''I can't believe you people!'' she exclaimed. ''Why aren't you taking aspirin?''

HOW ASPIRIN WORKS

In the late 1960s, the discovery that aspirin prolongs bleeding by inhibiting platelet aggregation started researchers down the path that eventually led to low-dose aspirin's use in heart attack prevention. But during the ensuing twenty-five years, researchers have learned a great deal more about how aspirin interferes with platelet aggregation. ADP, the chemical released by the platelets that was believed to trigger their aggregation, plays only a minor role in the process. In 1975, Swedish researchers identified the chemical primarily responsible—the prostaglandin, thromboxane-A_2.

Thromboxane plays a key role in the complex biochemical process known as the "coagulation cascade," which produces either a blood clot on the skin or a thrombus inside a blood vessel. When an artery or vein becomes injured, the cells at the injury site release a chemical called "arachidonic acid," a waxy substance that helps keep blood vessels flexible. An enzyme, cyclooxygenase, helps transform arachidonic acid into thromboxane-A_2, which triggers platelet aggregation. Aspirin has an antiprostaglandin effect. It deactivates cyclooxygenase and, as a result, inhibits the formation of thromboxane, thus impairing platelet aggregation and coronary artery thrombosis.

ASPIRIN BOOSTS SURVIVAL *DURING* HEART ATTACK

Of the nation's annual 1.5 million heart attacks, most of the 500,000 deaths occur within two hours after chest pain strikes. About twenty-five years ago, researchers began focusing on this critical 120-minute period. If, at the first sign of heart attack, coronary thrombosis could be quickly eliminated, heart attacks might be stopped before they could kill—and tens of thousands of lives could be saved. The key was to develop drugs that could rapidly dissolve (lyse) thrombi. Around the world, researchers began a quest for "thrombolytics."

Thrombolytic research did not make much headway until the 1980s, but in that decade remarkably effective thrombolytic drugs were developed. When administered in time, they prevent death and minimize heart damage in about 75 percent of cases. As this book goes to press, five have won FDA approval: streptokinase (Kabikinase, Streptase), tissue plasminogen activator (tPA, Activase), urokinase (Abbokinase), anistreplase (Eminase), and heparin (Liqaemin Sodium).

Thrombolytics have two major problems—availability and cost. To be effective, they must be administered as quickly as possible after the onset of chest pain. Unfortunately, thrombolytics are prescription drugs available only through emergency medical facilities. To benefit from them, heart attack sufferers must get to an emergency room—or have paramedics get to them—quickly, which is not always possible. In about 60 percent of heart attack deaths, the victim is dead on arrival at the hospital. In addition, thrombolytic drugs range in price from expensive to exorbitant. The two most widely used are streptokinase and tPA. The former costs about $200 per dose, the latter a whopping $2,000. An ideal thrombolytic would cost only pennies and be within arm's reach the moment chest pain begins. One is—aspirin. But like aspirin's other cardiovascular benefits, it took a while for this one to be appreciated.

The first investigation of aspirin as a thrombolytic was conducted in England during the late 1970s by the same Peter Elwood who'd headed two of the early aspirin-MI trials. He recruited British family physicians to administer either a placebo or 300 mg of aspirin as first-line treatment for patients the physicians believed were having heart attacks. Neither the physicians nor the patients knew who received the aspirin or placebo, so the trial was scientifically rigorous—prospective, randomized, double-blind, and placebo-controlled. A total of 1,705 heart attack sufferers (1,279 men and 426 women) were

followed for 29 days after receiving one of the two treatments. The death rates of the two groups were almost identical. "These results," Ellwood wrote in 1979 in the *Journal
of the Royal College of General Practitioners*, "give no en-
couragement to the use of aspirin in the early treatment of
myocardial infarction."

Nine years later, in 1983, *The Lancet* established aspirin
as an indispensible thrombolytic by publishing the findings of
the Second International Study of Infarct Survival, known as
ISIS-2. This ambitious, three-year effort involved 17,187
people admitted to 417 British hospitals with a diagnosis of
heart attack. They were randomized into four groups—placebo, one hour of intravenous streptokinase, one month of
low-dose aspirin (160 mg per day), and both streptokinase
and aspirin—and then followed for fifteen months. Compared
with the placebo treatment, both streptokinase alone and aspirin alone produced significant reductions in deaths from heart
attack—25 percent and 23 percent, respectively. Together,
the two treatments had a synergistic effect, reducing deaths
42 percent. Some patients were not treated for as long as
twenty-four hours after their chest pain began, but even in
this late-treatment group, the two drugs alone and together
saved many lives—21 percent fewer deaths among those taking streptokinase alone, 21 percent fewer for aspirin alone,
and 38 percent fewer for the two drugs combined. Aspirin
treatment also produced significant reductions in stroke and
subsequent heart attack during the follow-up period.

The ISIS-2 researchers concluded that physicians using
streptokinase should switch to a combination of the drug plus
aspirin. For the public, they strongly endorsed aspirin as first-
aid for suspicious chest pain. Unlike streptokinase and other
thrombolytics,

> aspirin does not require particularly careful monitoring, and
> it might well be appropriate to start it as soon as possible,
> provided there are no clear contraindications. The side effects

of low-dose aspirin seem negligible and the drug costs are small. Aspirin could be widely used not only in developed countries but also in countries with limited medical resources. If one month of low-dose aspirin were given to 1 million new [heart attack] patients per year, then tens of thousands of deaths, reinfarctions, and strokes could be avoided or substantially delayed. And these benefits could be doubled if low-dose aspirin were continued for at least a few years.

Other studies have shown that aspirin treatment also enhances the thrombolytic effectiveness of tPA. And a 1991 meta-analysis in the *Journal of Clinical Epidemiology,* which combined the results of several thrombolytic trials, showed that the death rate reductions achieved with streptokinase and tPA alone almost doubled with the addition of aspirin.

Unfortunately, most thrombolytic studies have investigated these drugs when administered in hospitals. They have not dealt with first aid for suspected heart attack, which is considerably more important given the substantial proportion of victims who die before they reach hospitals. Recently, two U.S. Army physicians decried this oversight in a letter to *The Lancet:*

Aspirin . . . rivals the [other] thrombolytic agents. [It] has a demonstrable antiplatelet effect within five minutes. We propose the earliest possible use of aspirin in the face of [suspected heart attack] chest pain. The [immediate] use of aspirin by the public in the minutes to hours before [obtaining] medical attention has the potential to thwart thrombus development, delay infarction, reduce sudden death outside hospitals, and further improve the prospects of patients who reach hospitals. The risk of [such] one-time aspirin use seems very small.

In case of suspected heart attack, physicians recommend taking regular aspirin, not the enteric-coated variety. Enteric coatings seal the drug under a protective layer that prevents stomach upset but also delays its absorption into the blood-stream. Regular aspirin reaches peak blood levels within thirty minutes. Enteric-coated brands take about sixty minutes. The key to thrombolytic intervention in heart attack is speed, so in the vast majority of cases, it would be unwise to delay absorption. For even faster absorption, crush the tablet and mix it with water.

ASPIRIN, HEART ATTACK, AND WOMEN

Heart attack is the number one killer of American women, but until quite recently women were an afterthought in heart disease research. The vast majority of studies either excluded women or used only token numbers. This oversight is now being rectified as researchers have come to appreciate coronary artery disease's deadly toll on women:

• Since 1950, the incidence of heart disease has declined in men but risen in women (largely because so many women took up smoking).
• Of the nation's 500,000 heart attack deaths each year, 48 percent—about 240,000—occur among women.
• More women die from heart disease than from *all cancers combined.*
• Unlike men, few women suffer heart attacks before age 50. The female sex hormone, estrogen, apparently protects them. After menopause, when the estrogen level falls, women's risk of heart attack soars.
• More than half of adult women have cholesterol levels above 200 mg/dl. In women, high cholesterol often begins in the teens.
• About 10 percent of women over age 45 have some form of cardiovascular disease.
• About half of women over 55 have high blood pressure. Among women over 65, the figure is 67 percent.

• Doctors tend to take chest pain more seriously in men than in women.

• Finally, doctors tend to treat heart attack more aggressively in men than in women. A larger proportion of men are referred for coronary artery bypass surgery. Physicians' wait-and-see attitude toward women heart attack survivors may be one reason why during the year after a heart attack only 31 percent of men die compared with 39 percent of women.

Only half of the early aspirin–heart attack clinical trials included any women, and in the German-Austrian trial, aspirin reduced heart attack risk only in men, not in women. Researchers speculated that even if aspirin helped men, it probably wouldn't help women because of the two genders' different levels of sex hormones. Men have more testosterone in their bloodstreams, women have more estrogen. Estrogen has complicated effects on the female cardiovascular system. In general, it protects against heart attack until menopause, but the extra estrogen in birth control pills tends to increase blood clotting and thrombosis, especially in women who smoke. Testosterone, on the other hand, increases aspirin's antiplatelet effect. Conclusion: Aspirin should only help those in whom testosterone predominates, in other words, men, not women.

Harvard's Joann E. Manson thought otherwise, and investigated aspirin's effect on women's risk of heart attack using the Nurses' Health Study, a six-year (1980–86), prospective, observational project that surveyed the life-styles and health habits—including aspirin consumption—of 87,678 American nurses aged thirty-four to sixty-five who, at the project's inception, had not had cancer, stroke, or heart attack. Compared with the nurses who consumed no aspirin, those who took one to six tablets a week suffered significantly fewer first heart attacks—25 percent fewer overall, and 32 percent fewer for the nurses over 50. Taking more than six aspirins a week did not reduce risk further. An editorial accompanying Manson's 1991 report in the *Journal of the American Medical Association* called the findings "intriguing," but hastened to warn that survey-based studies do not carry the scientific weight of rigorous clinical trials. The next logical step, the journal said, was a women's version of the Physicians' Health Study.

That study was launched later in 1991, with a $17 million grant from NIH. The Women's Health Study has enrolled approximately 40,000 nurses over 50 who have no history of cancer or cardiovascular disease. Using a prospective, randomized, double-blind, placebo-controlled design, the researchers plan to study not only aspirin use for the prevention of heart attack and stroke, but also supplementation with vitamin E and beta-carotene (a form of vitamin A) for prevention of cancer. Participants are scheduled to be followed from 1992 through 1997, and the results should be published within two years after that.

Meanwhile, the question of aspirin's ability to reduce heart attack risk in women remains open. So far, the evidence appears positive.

THAT "HEARTBURN" MAY ACTUALLY BE A HEART ATTACK

An estimated 10 to 20 percent of Americans—some 25 to 50 million people—regularly suffer the burning, belching, and regurgitation of bitter stomach acids misnamed "heartburn." Actually, heartburn has nothing to do with the heart. The burning feeling in the chest is caused by a valve malfunction at the top of the stomach. The valve doesn't stay closed as it should. When it remains open, caustic stomach acids splash up the esophagus, the tube that carries food down from the throat. It's the esophagus that gets burned, not the heart. In addition to its burning sensation, episodes of what many people dismiss as heartburn may cause chest pain so severe that they sometimes fear they're having a heart attack. The fact is, *sometimes they are.*

Heart attacks don't always make people clutch their chests and keel over. Frequently, people having heart attacks dismiss their chest pain as "just heartburn." But that "heartburn" may be a heart attack if the chest pain occurs along with any of the following symptoms:

- Pain that radiates up under the jaw, or out to either shoulder or arm (more commonly, the left arm)
- Unusual sweating
- Nausea
- Shortness of breath
- Dizziness

If you or anyone you know experiences heartburn with any of these other symptoms for more than ten minutes:

- Call 911. Don't delay. People suffering "heartburn" heart attacks often dismiss as ridiculous the idea that their chest symptoms might be serious. Don't take "no" for an answer. If you're wrong, you'll both laugh about it later. If you're right, you might save a life.
- Tell the 911 operator: "Suspected heart attack." Give your location and summarize the symptoms.
- Ask the 911 operator about the advisability of giving the person aspirin immediately. Its thrombolytic effect improves the likelihood of survival. And if the chest pain really is heartburn, the risk of side effects is small. Heart attack sufferers sometimes have trouble swallowing. Assess the situation with the help of the 911 operator.
- Wait for instructions. Don't hang up until the operator does. You may be instructed to wait for an ambulance or take the person to an emergency medical facility.

While waiting for the ambulance, or on the way to the emergency room, make the person as comfortable as possible. Loosen tight collars and any constricting clothing. For nausea, have the person lie down. But don't give any food or drink, except for a sip of water if the 911 operator advises giving the person aspirin. Choking is possible, although for most people the benefit of giving aspirin outweighs the risk of choking. Talk to the person; reassure him or her that if it is a heart attack, survival chances are very good with prompt emergency medical attention. Reassurance is crucial. Heart attack sufferers often panic, which places additional strain on their already-damaged hearts.

Sometimes, after rushing to the emergency room, you learn that the suspected heart attack was, in fact, heartburn. Try not to feel embarrassed. Plenty of physicians experience particularly strong heartburn and become convinced *they* are having heart attacks. It's better to be safe than sorry, especially if the person has any heart disease risk factors: smoking, obesity, diabetes, high blood pressure, high cholesterol, sedentary life-style, Type-A behavior, and/or a personal or family history of heart disease.

ASPIRIN HELPS CONTROL ANGINA

The severe chest pain of angina (medically known as myocardial ischemia, literally, lack of blood flow to the heart wall) is a symptom of a malnourished heart. As atherosclerotic plaques decrease blood flow through the coronary arteries, the heart does not receive all the food and oxygen it needs and the result is chest pain. In stable angina, pain occurs only during physical exertion. As the condition becomes severe (unstable angina), chest pain occurs even while at rest. America's six-million angina sufferers are prime candidates for heart attacks.

Beginning in the early 1980s, researchers showed that in unstable angina the coronary arteries become narrowed not only by atherosclerotic plaques but also by thrombi not quite large enough to trigger heart attack. It didn't take long for researchers to try aspirin as a treatment.

The first major success was the 1983 Veterans Administration Cooperative Study mentioned earlier in this chapter. Its 1,266 male subjects with unstable angina took a daily dose of either a placebo or 324 mg of aspirin (one standard tablet). After twelve weeks, the aspirin group suffered 51 percent fewer fatal and 51 percent fewer nonfatal heart attacks.

These results have been repeatedly corroborated. In 1985, Canadian researchers randomized 555 men and women hospitalized with unstable angina into four groups: placebo, aspirin (325 mg, one standard tablet), another antiplatelet drug, and both drugs. Participants took their medication four times a day for two years. Compared with the placebo group, the aspirin users had 51 percent fewer heart attacks, a highly significant result. (The other antiplatelet drug showed no benefit.) As for gastrointestinal side effects, the aspirin group reported problems only slightly more frequently than those taking the placebo. "Patients of either sex who are hospitalized with unstable angina are likely to benefit from . . . aspirin," the researchers concluded in the *New England Journal of Medicine.* "We estimate that in the U.S., perhaps 500,000 people per year enter coronary care units with unstable angina. There is a sizable population for whom aspirin would offer considerable benefit."

The most recent trial, a 1991 Swedish study involving 796 men with unstable angina, showed significant benefit with even less aspirin—just 75 mg a day (about one-quarter of a standard tablet). After one year, the aspirin group experienced 48 percent fewer heart attacks and a substantial reduction in angina symptoms. At such a low aspirin dose, fewer than 4 percent of the aspirin users complained of gastrointestinal side effects. "With aspirin, the reductions of MI, angina, and death were impressive and side effects were rare," the researchers wrote in the *Journal of the American College of Cardiology.* "At this dose, aspirin is extremely inexpensive and treatment is very cost-effective. Low-dose aspirin treatment should start as soon as possible and continue for at least three months after an episode of unstable angina provided there are no absolute contraindictions. Continuous treatment for a longer period should be considered.''

What about less severe stable angina? In 1991, using data from the Physicians' Health Study, Harvard researchers discovered significant benefit. The landmark study of aspirin and heart attack included 333 men with stable angina but no history of heart attack or stroke. Compared with those in the placebo group, stable angina sufferers who took aspirin suffered 30 percent fewer heart attacks. "Patients with chronic stable angina are at high risk for cardiovascular death," the researchers wrote in *Annals of Internal Medicine.* "Alternate-day aspirin therapy greatly reduced their risk of first MI."

ASPIRIN IMPROVES BYPASS SURGERY RESULTS

One standard treatment for severe angina or heart attack is coronary artery bypass grafting (CABG), also called "cardiac revascularization" and popularly known as bypass surgery. According to the American Heart Association, 368,000 bypass operations are performed in the U.S. each year, about three-quarters involving men over 45. Bypass surgery involves snipping a section of blood vessel from another part of the body (usually the leg or chest) and using it to create a detour around the blocked section of a coronary artery. While sometimes a lifesaving procedure, CABG usually provides only temporary benefit because, over time, the grafted blood vessel tends to become as blocked as the one it replaced, increasing risk of heart attack and often necessitating another costly bypass.

In a 1991 report in the journal *Circulation,* Australian surgeons evaluated aspirin treatment of bypass patients starting immediately after surgery. The surgeons took a risk giving their patients aspirin because it prolongs bleeding, and bleeding is a potentially serious complication of *any* surgery. Fortunately, the aspirin treatment did not increase postsurgical blood loss significantly—and it produced major benefits. One year after the bypasses, the researchers used special X-rays to determine the extent of blockage in the grafted blood vessels. Compared with controls, the aspirin group showed only half as much blockage. These findings must be corroborated before they can be considered compelling, but postbypass aspirin treatment may well reduce risk of heart attack after bypass surgery and increase graft-vessel life, reducing the need for repeat surgery.

ASPIRIN IMPROVES ANGIOPLASTY RESULTS

A newer, less invasive, less costly treatment for severe coronary artery disease is percutaneous transluminal coronary angioplasty (PTCA), often called "balloon angioplasty" or simply "angioplasty." The physician inserts a narrow tube (catheter) into an artery in an arm or leg and, guided by X-ray images, threads it into the obstructed coronary artery. Once it's in place, a second catheter with a balloon tip is threaded through the first. When the balloon reaches the blockage, the physician inflates it and compresses the plaque, enlarging the artery so that blood can flow more easily to the heart. The problem with angioplasty is that in about 25 percent of cases, the newly unblocked artery clogs up again (restenosis), usually within six months. Then the options are more angioplasty or bypass surgery.

Since angioplasty was introduced in 1977, various antiplatelet drugs, including aspirin, have been used in an effort to prevent restenosis—without much success. But in 1988, a Canadian study showed that while the combination of aspirin (330 mg, about one standard tablet, three times a day) and dipyridamole (Persantine), another antiplatelet drug, did not prevent restenosis, it significantly reduced heart attacks within 14 hours of the procedure. "Patients undergoing angioplasty," the researchers concluded in the *New England Journal of Medicine*, "should follow an antiplatelet regimen from 24 hours before until at least 48 hours afterward to reduce the incidence of [angioplasty-related] myocardial infarction."

Then, in 1991, Australian researchers showed that low-dose aspirin does indeed help reduce restenosis after angioplasty. They divided 212 angioplasty patients into placebo and aspirin groups (110 mg a day, about one-third of a standard tablet) and followed them for six months. Significant restenosis occurred in 38 percent of the placebo group, but in just 25 percent of the aspirin users, a modest but significant difference. Postangioplasty aspirin treatment, the researchers wrote in the *American Journal of Cardiology*, "has a small beneficial effect" on prevention of restenosis.

NOT BY ASPIRIN ALONE

As miraculous as aspirin may be in reducing the risk of heart attack and angina, regular low-dose aspirin use is *no substitute* for controlling the heart disease risk factors.

If you smoke, quit. Quitting helps at any age. Risk of heart attack immediately begins to decline. After five years as an ex-smoker, a person's risk drops about 40 percent. Ten years after quitting, ex-smokers' heart attack risk approaches that of lifelong nonsmokers. For help quitting, ask your physician. (See Bibliography for recommended reading.)

Control your blood pressure. For every six-point decrease in diastolic pressure (the second number in a blood pressure reading), risk of heart attack declines about 10 percent and risk of stroke drops 40 percent. Although a tendency to hypertension can be inherited (especially among African Americans), moderately elevated blood pressure can often be reduced through weight loss, regular moderate exercise, a low-salt (low-sodium) diet, and stress management. If necessary, several drug treatments are available by prescription.

Reduce your cholesterol. Every 1 percent decrease in total cholesterol produces about a 2 percent reduction in heart attack risk. The best way to reduce cholesterol is to eat less fat. In the typical American diet, 40 percent of calories come from fat. To lower cholesterol, less than 30 percent of calories should come from fat, and the lower the fat content of one's diet, the better. A low-fat diet means eating more fiber—not just oat bran but all whole-grain products—beans, and fresh fruits and vegetables. Studies show that a diet high in garlic also reduces cholesterol. In addition to a low-fat diet, regular exercise helps increase HDL levels. (See Bibliography for recommended reading.)

Another way to reduce cholesterol is to take niacin, also known as vitamin B_3 or nicotinic acid. (Nicotinic acid has some structural similarity to the nicotine found in cigarette smoke but none of its damaging effects.) In doses ranging from 1,200 to 2,000 mg a day, niacin has been shown to cut cholesterol by as much as 22 percent. However, at doses high enough to reduce cholesterol, niacin also causes an unpleasant side effect, "niacin flush," a reddening, burning, itching, tingling sensation in the face, neck, arms, and upper chest. Niacin flush occurs because the vitamin acts as a vasodilator and opens the skin's blood vessels. The extra blood near the skin surface causes the reddening and other odd sensations. Niacin flush is not dangerous, but it can be frightening and annoying. Fortunately, researchers at the Medical University of South Carolina have reported a way to reduce the reddening and warmth of niacin flush (but not the itching and tingling): Thirty minutes before taking niacin, take one standard aspirin tablet. Anyone taking niacin to reduce cholesterol (or aspirin then niacin) should do so in consultation with a physician.

If you're overweight, lose those extra pounds.
But don't get sucked in by the latest fad diet. Diets don't work. Lose weight gradually—no more than one pound a week—through a combination of regular, moderate exercise and a low-fat, low-cholesterol, high-fiber diet. (See Bibliography for recommended reading.)

Enjoy regular moderate exercise.
You don't have to sweat buckets to gain health benefits from exercise. Studies show that adults who have not exercised in years gain significant protection against heart disease by walking just two miles at a moderate pace three times a week. Two miles may sound daunting, but it's only a few circuits around most malls. Almost anyone can take walks, bike, swim, dance, or garden, all of which provide cardiovascular benefits. But if you have any of the heart disease risk factors, check with your physician before starting an exercise program.

Change your Type-A behavior to Type-B.
The first step is to assess your stress load with StressMap™ Self-Assessment Questionnaire. (To obtain the questionnaire, send $16.95 to Essi Systems, Inc., 126 South Park, San Francisco, CA 94107; [415] 541-4911.) It takes about an hour to answer the twenty-one-question sets and to plot your results on the ingenious scoring grid. Once completed, the scoring grid shows at a glance where your stress problems and coping strengths lie. Then incorporate any stress-reducing activities you enjoy into your life, among them: yoga, meditation, exercise, gardening, family time, music, hobbies, prayer, talking with friends, volunteer work, and/or playing with a pet.

Many heart attack–prevention programs now include components specifically designed to help harried Type-As evolve into more mellow, less frenzied Type Bs. Helpful steps include: spending more time with friends and family, never interrupting anyone, saying no to business and social opportunities unless you're likely to remember them five years later, developing hobbies and other interests outside of work, and watching someone struggle with a task you know you could do faster and better—and not intervening.

Consider a contraceptive other than the Pill. If you have heart disease risk factors, ask your physician or family planning provider about the advisability of switching to another method.

CHAPTER TWO

ASPIRIN HELPS PREVENT
STROKE AND SENILITY

In late 1991, researchers studying aspirin for stroke prevention embraced a new concept: less, much less. Two studies published almost simultaneously showed that as little as *one-tenth of a standard aspirin tablet* a day provided the same protection as the much larger doses considered the stroke-prevention standard since the late 1980s. One study, a three-year Swedish trial published in *The Lancet,* showed that compared with the placebo group, those taking just 75 mg of aspirin a day (one-quarter of a standard tablet) suffered 18 percent fewer strokes, a reduction almost identical to the results achieved using higher doses. The other, a three-year Dutch trial published in the *New England Journal of Medicine,* showed that an ultralow 30 mg a day prevented stroke just as well as a dose nine times greater. The question, the researchers wrote, was no longer *how much* aspirin was necessary to prevent tens of thousands of stroke each year but *how little*.

A BLOW TO THE HEAD

More than three hundred years ago, physicians noticed a disturbing pattern. Some people who'd not been struck on the head reported sudden severe head pain, as though they'd been bludgeoned, and soon afterward collapsed either dead or seriously disabled. The ailment occurred suddenly, like a "stroke of bad luck," so they named it after the word then used for any sudden unexpected event, stroke.

Like heart attack, stroke is a cardiovascular disease, but the affected arteries are located in the brain. Stroke is the nation's third leading cause of death (after heart disease and cancer). Americans suffer about 500,000 strokes each year and 150,000 stroke deaths. Approximately three million living Americans have had strokes. Some recover fully, but many suffer permanent disabilities.

Stroke deaths, like those from heart attack, have declined substantially in recent years—more than 30 percent since 1979. Authorities credit improved treatment of high blood pressure, the leading stroke risk factor. Yet stroke remains a major killer despite the decline in deaths.

A stroke occurs when an artery in the head becomes either blocked or ruptured and can't deliver oxygen and nutrients to part of the brain. Deprived of nourishment for just a few minutes, the nerve cells in the affected area die. At the same time, the body parts those cells control become impaired, causing such stroke-related disabilities as paralysis, vision or speech difficulties, or an inability to recognize loved ones.

There are four major types of stroke, two caused by blocked

blood flow (ischemia), and two by ruptured blood vessels that bleed (hemorrhage). The first two, cerebral thrombosis and cerebral embolism, together known as ischemic stroke, account for about 80 percent of strokes. The later two, cerebral hemorrhage and subarachnoid hemorrhage, collectively hemorrhagic stroke, occur much less frequently but are considerably more likely to be fatal.

Cerebral thrombosis is by far the leading cause of stroke, accounting for about 65 percent of what physicians call "cerebrovascular events" ("cerebro" means "brain," "vascular" refers to the blood vessels). Cerebral thrombosis, also known as ischemic brain infarction, is the result of atherosclerosis, the same narrowing of the arteries that causes heart attack. Cerebral thrombosis often occurs at night or first thing in the morning when blood pressure is naturally low, which increases risk of arterial blockage by internal blood clots (thrombi). Just as many heart attacks are preceded by angina, about 10 percent of thrombotic strokes are preceded by ministrokes known as transient ischemic attacks (TIAs). TIAs occur when a thrombus temporarily blocks an artery in the brain, causing a brief period of substantially reduced blood flow, or ischemia. TIA symptoms—numbness, faintness, dizziness, clumsiness, and/or loss of speech or vision, particularly in one eye—strike suddenly and usually don't last more than five minutes (although some last up to twenty-four hours). TIAs are the most predictive risk factor for cerebral thrombosis, multiplying risk tenfold. About one-third of those who experience a TIA have a stroke within five years. Half of post-TIA strokes occur within a year, 20 percent strike within one month. TIAs also double the risk of heart attack.

Cerebral embolism, which accounts for about 17 percent of strokes, occurs when an embolus, an abnormal traveler in the bloodstream, lodges in an artery in the brain and blocks blood flow. Most cerebral emboli are thrombi formed in the heart when its two smaller chambers, the atria, quiver instead of beating normally (atrial fibrillation). Instead of being pumped out of the heart as it would if the atria beat properly, some blood pools in these chambers, and eventually coagulates into a thrombus, which is termed an embolus if it leaves the heart. An estimated two million Americans suffer atrial fibrillation, and about 15 percent of strokes occur in people with this heart problem. The risk of strokes associated with atrial fibrillation increases dramatically with age. At fifty, only 2 percent of strokes are related to atrial fibrillation, by eighty the figure is 24 percent.

About 10 percent of strokes are caused by cerebral hemorrhage, which occurs when an artery in the brain bursts, flooding part of the organ with blood. The cause is usually an aneurysm, a weak spot in a blood vessel, rather like a bald spot on a tire. Just as the combination of a bald spot and increased air pressure can blow out a tire, the combination of a cerebral aneurysm and high blood pressure can cause cerebral hemorrhage.

Subarachnoid hemorrhage accounts for about 8 percent of strokes. A blood vessel on the surface of the brain ruptures, spilling blood into the area between the brain and the skull (subarachnoid space).

In both types of hemorrhagic stroke, brain damage is related to the amount of bleeding. In about half the cases, profuse bleeding causes so much pressure on the brain that the person dies. In contrast, only about 25 percent of those who suffer ischemic strokes die.

Compared with ischemic stroke survivors, those who survive hemorrhagic strokes generally fare better. Ischemic strokes kill part of the brain, making recovery difficult. In hemorrhagic strokes, the part of the brain near the rupture is less likely to die. Once the pressure caused by the hemorrhage has been relieved, the brain is often able to at least recover partially.

Like heart disease, stroke has several risk factors, some of which can be controlled, while others cannot. The ones beyond our control include:

Heredity. Like heart disease, stroke tends to run in families. The closer the blood relative(s), the higher the risk.

Age. Stroke can strike at any age, though it's rare until age 30. More than 70 percent of strokes strike Americans over 65.

Gender. Men are more likely to have strokes than women. Among those over sixty-five, men suffer 9 percent more strokes than women. Among those under sixty-five, men suffer 48 percent more.

Race. Compared with the white population, African Americans are 50 percent more likely to have strokes, and considerably more likely to suffer stroke-related disability. Most experts link African Americans' elevated stroke risk with their unusually high rate of high blood pressure.

Diabetes. Diabetes increases risk of all cardiovascular diseases. The diabetics at highest risk for stroke are those with high blood pressure. Diabetes increases stroke risk more for women than for men.

Prior stroke. Compared to those who have never had strokes, those who have face many times the risk of having another, although men's risk of recurrent stroke is greater than women's.

Carotid bruit. A bruit is an abnormal sound in an artery that a doctor can detect with a stethoscope. A carotid bruit is an abnormal sound in the carotid artery in the neck, which supplies blood to the brain. Carotid bruits suggest significant atherosclerosis and increased risk for stroke.

Stroke risk factors that can be changed include:

High blood pressure (hypertension). Hypertension is the most important risk factor for stroke. The higher one's blood pressure, the greater one's risk. For more information, see the discussion of high blood pressure and heart disease in Chapter 1.

Smoking. See the discussion in Chapter 1.

Elevated cholesterol. See the discussion in Chapter 1.

Heart disease. Independent of other risk factors, people with heart disease have about double the average risk of stroke.

Transient ischemic attacks. Although only about 10 percent of strokes are preceded by these ministrokes, TIAs are a clear signal of substantial stroke risk.

Several other odd risk factors also contribute to stroke:

Geography. For reasons that remain a mystery, the Southeast is the nation's "Stroke Belt": Alabama, Arkansas, Georgia, Kentucky, Louisiana, Mississippi, the Carolinas, Tennessee, and Virginia. These states have large populations of African Americans who are at increased risk, but many Northeastern and Midwest states also have large African-American populations and are not part of the Stroke Belt.

Weather. Stroke deaths occur more often during periods of very hot or cold weather.

Income. More than heart attack, stroke is associated with poverty.

In recent years, significant progress has been made in stroke rehabilitation. Studies have shown that the faster rehabilitation efforts begin, the greater the chance of significant improvement, even in cases of severely disabling stroke. Still, stroke remains a major cause of disability.

Fortunately, in people who have had TIAs or minor strokes, aspirin reduces subsequent stroke risk by approximately 25 percent.

LATER START, EARLIER SUCCESS

Like their colleagues in heart attack research, stroke researchers became quite excited when aspirin was shown to have antiplatelet and, presumably, antithrombotic effects. After all, about 80 percent of strokes are caused by thrombotic (or embolic) arterial blockage. Stroke researchers were also intrigued by the rheumatoid arthritis autopsy study (discussed in Chapter 1), which showed a noticeable, though statistically insignificant, reduction in ischemic stroke among rheumatoid arthritis sufferers, who typically take a great deal of aspirin. But the only scientifically persuasive way to test aspirin as a stroke preventive was through costly prospective, randomized, placebo-controlled, double-blind clinical trials.

Funding such studies was difficult enough for heart disease investigators even though heart attack accounts for 23 percent of U.S. deaths. As deadly and disabling as stroke can be, by comparison, it's a smaller public health problem: "only" 500,000 strokes a year, 150,000 deaths—7 percent of the nation's mortality. In addition, cardiologists, who deal with heart attack, have historically been more politically powerful in government research-funding agencies than neurologists, who deal with stroke. Funding for aspirin–heart attack studies came slowly; for aspirin-stroke studies, it was glacial.

Eventually, six major aspirin-stroke trials were published,

plus fifteen smaller, less ambitious studies. In 1977, when the first appeared in the journal *Stroke* (three years after publication of the first aspirin–heart attack trial, and two years after the start of the $17 million AMIS trial), it buoyed stroke researchers and heart disease investigators alike because, in marked contrast to the heart attack studies published until that time, the initial aspirin-stroke trial showed statistically significant benefit.

This trial was a three-year project coordinated by researchers at the University of Texas Health Science Center in Houston. They had to grapple with the same problem their heart disease colleagues faced, namely, how to hold costs down while at the same time enrolling enough participants to have a reasonable chance of discovering a significant difference between the aspirin and control groups. They decided to focus on those at highest risk for ischemic stroke, people who had already had at least one TIA. The researchers divided a relatively small number of subjects, 178 men and women from 45 to 75, into the usual two groups. Twice a day, one group received a placebo, the other group 650 mg of aspirin (two standard tablets). The aspirin group suffered 38 percent fewer strokes, but small numbers—thirteen strokes in the aspirin group, nineteen in the placebo group—made the difference statistically insignificant. Among participants who had had multiple TIAs before enrolling in the study, aspirin produced a significant reduction in stroke risk. The researchers cautiously suggested that perhaps the drug should be recommended to those who'd had multiple TIAs. An editorial accompanying the study was more effusive, touting the frequency of multiple TIAs and the "marked reduction" in strokes in the aspirin group. As for side effects, the placebo takers reported almost as many upset stomachs as the aspirin users. Despite this study's limitations, aspirin looked both safe and effective as a stroke preventive. The aspirin-stroke score read: one study pro, zero con.

The second stroke trial was published the following year

by Canadian researchers. This two-year study divided 585 men and women who'd had previous TIAs into four groups: one group took a placebo, one took aspirin (one standard tablet four times a day), one took another anticoagulant drug, and one took both drugs. The other anticoagulant showed no benefit, but compared with the placebo group, the aspirin takers suffered a statistically significant 31 percent fewer strokes. The benefits, however, accrued only to men: When the aspirin group was divided by sex, the women experienced no benefit, while the men's stroke risk fell 48 percent. At a time when aspirin looked like a bust for heart attack prevention, the Canadian researchers wrote in the *New England Journal of Medicine:* "Aspirin's highly significant [stroke-preventive] benefit leaves little doubt that it is truly efficacious in men." The researchers concluded, "It would be reasonable to recommend that men with TIAs or minor strokes who are able to tolerate aspirin should take it." The score was now: two studies pro, zero con.

In an editorial the following month, the journal *Stroke* could barely contain its enthusiasm: "Male patients threatened with stroke will benefit by daily use of one of the oldest and commonest pharmaceutical agents—aspirin. . . . [The Canadian study results] demand the attention of all [physicians] engaged in clinical practice. [Aspirin's] effectiveness in women has not been established. Men, on the other hand, will benefit."

The third and fourth aspirin-stroke trials were published simultaneously in 1983. One, by a Danish team, was a two-year study of 203 men and women, average age 60, with histories of previous TIAs. Half received a placebo, the other half, 1,000 mg of aspirin a day (about three standard tablets). Aspirin produced no reduction in stroke risk. In fact, the aspirin group suffered *more* strokes than the placebo group, but that finding was not statistically significant.

The accompanying study, by a French team, was a three-year study of 604 men and women with a history of TIAs, most in their 50s and 60s. One-third received a placebo, one-third received 1,000 mg of aspirin a day (three standard tablets), and one-third received the same amount of aspirin plus another anticoagulant drug. The other drug made no difference, but compared with the placebo takers, those in the aspirin groups suffered 42 percent fewer strokes, a significant difference. Unlike the previous studies, there were no sex differences—aspirin helped the women as much as the men. About 9 percent of the aspirin users reported abdominal pain and 1.5 percent developed ulcers. The researchers suggested that their 1,000-mg aspirin dose may have been higher than necessary: "It has been suggested that doses of aspirin as low as 150 mg every two or three days [might] produce inhibition of thrombosis." But even at their high dose, the researchers considered the side effects in their study a small price to pay for such a major reduction in stroke risk: "These side effects . . . certainly did not outweigh the benefit of aspirin." All that remained, they concluded, was to determine the optimal stroke-preventive aspirin dose.

In an accompanying editorial, neurologist Mark Dyken of the University of Indiana School of Medicine accused the Danish team of commiting a Type II error, failing to discover a real effect and concluding mistakenly that it does not exist. The main cause of Type II errors is small sample size, the same problem that bedeviled the early aspirin–heart attack trials. With just 203 subjects, the Danish trial couldn't confirm what the three other trials had all determined—aspirin helps prevent stroke in those at high risk. "This critique is not intended to single out [the Danish study] as having more defects than the others . . . ," but the *Stroke* editorial certainly read that way. By 1983, *Stroke*'s editors were clearly sold on aspirin. The score was now: three studies solidly pro, one con (but flawed).

The fifth aspirin-stroke trial, published in 1987, was the European Stroke Prevention Study (ESPS), an ambitious cooperative effort among researchers at sixteen medical centers in Belgium, Denmark, Ireland, Finland, Holland, and Britain. The ESPS investigators enrolled 2,500 men and women with a history of TIAs and gave half a placebo and half 325 mg of aspirin (one standard tablet) three times a day plus another antiplatelet drug. Two years later, the aspirin group had suffered 33 percent fewer strokes. Not surprisingly, the aspirin group reported more stomach pain and ulcers and, oddly, more headaches. But as the largest aspirin-stroke study ever, four times larger than its biggest predecessor, the ESPS trial provided more convincing evidence than ever that aspirin prevented stroke in those at high risk. The score was now: four studies pro, one con (but flawed).

Soon after, in 1988, came the sixth aspirin-stroke study, the U.K.-TIA trial. This large British effort enrolled 2,435 men and women, average age sixty, who'd had TIAs. One-third took a placebo, one-third received 600 mg of aspirin (somewhat less than two standard tablets) twice a day, and one-third took 300 mg of aspirin (slightly less than one standard tablet) once a day. After four years, the two aspirin groups showed 18 percent fewer strokes, a significant benefit, but only 7 percent fewer stroke deaths, which was not significant. The lower dose of aspirin (300 mg a day) was as effective as the higher dose (1,200 mg) but caused only a fraction of the side effects. Writing in the *British Medical Journal,* the researchers expressed "frustration" that their large, long-term study showed no significant decrease in stroke deaths with daily aspirin treatment. But in combination with the other five trials, they said, the evidence "shows conclusively" that aspirin helps prevent stroke. The final score was: five studies significantly pro, one con (but flawed).

By 1988, when the U.K.-TIA trial was published, meta-analysis, had been accepted, and the same issue of the *British Medical Journal* included a meta-analysis of thirteen aspirin-stroke trials—the six major studies discussed here and seven others that were too small or too brief to stand alone. The statisticians calculated that aspirin reduced stroke risk 22 percent: "The most convenient and least expensive antiplatelet agent is low-dose aspirin."

Three years later, in 1991, a team of Canadian biostatisticians published another meta-analysis of the six major aspirin-stroke trials discussed above: "Aspirin alone produced an 18 percent decrease in all strokes," a figure slightly lower than the one in the earlier meta-analysis. The Canadian researchers attributed the difference to their more complete elimination of the effects of the other antiplatelet drugs used in several of the trials. Although their numbers came out slightly different, their conclusion in the *Family Practice Research Journal* was the same: "These results support the use of aspirin as a first-line treatment for the prevention of ischemic events in patients with TIAs and minor strokes."

That same year, another study provided persuasive evidence that aspirin helps prevent not only the kind of ischemic stroke associated with TIA, cerebral thrombosis, but cerebral embolism as well. As previously noted, cerebral embolism is often preceded by atrial fibrillation, quivering of the heart's small chambers. Atrial fibrillation increases risk of cerebral embolism sixfold. In this study of 1,330 people with atrial fibrillation, one-third were given a placebo, one-third 325 mg of aspirin a day (one standard tablet), and one-third another anticoagulant, the prescription drug warfarin. Warfarin prevented the most strokes and stroke deaths, but compared with the placebo group, the aspirin users experienced 42 percent fewer cerebral embolisms and 32 percent fewer embolic stroke deaths. Writing in the journal *Circulation,* the researchers concluded: "Patients with atrial fibrillation who can safely take aspirin or warfarin should [do so] to reduce risk of stroke."

THE RIGHT DOSE

By the end of 1991, the issue was settled. Aspirin helped prevent both kinds of ischemic stroke. But three questions remained:

- What was the optimal dose?
- Does aspirin prevent stroke in women?
- And in the wake of the Physicians' Health Study showing that the drug prevents first heart attacks in healthy people, does aspirin prevent first strokes in those with no history of TIAs or atrial fibrillation?

As this book goes to press, researchers speculate that aspirin helps prevent first strokes in the healthy population, but no study of the question has been published.

The other two questions, however, have been answered. Regarding optimal dose, a mere 30 mg of aspirin a day (less than one-tenth of a standard tablet) prevented stroke as well as 283 mg in the 1991 Dutch TIA trial. This study enrolled 3,131 men and women with previous TIAs and followed them for two and a half years. Half took the ultralow dose; half took the higher dose (which was lower than the dose used in any of the six major trials). In the 283 mg group, 15.2 percent had a stroke. In the 30 mg group, the figure was 14.7 percent. Although major bleeding complications occurred about equally in both groups, other expected aspirin side effects—stomach distress and gastrointestinal bleeding—occurred 17 percent less frequently in the ultralow-dose group. The journal *Family Practice* editorialized: "In medicine, more is not always better. If a low drug dose is as effective as [a higher one] in preventing stroke, the lower complication rate argues for its use."

Unfortunately, as of 1991, many physicians still do not prescribe daily aspirin to patients with a history of TIAs, according to a survey published in *Archives of Internal Medicine*. Researchers at Long Island Jewish Medical Center mailed a questionnaire to 480 physician-professors at two university medical centers: Only 64 percent routinely prescribed aspirin to those who'd had TIAs.

ASPIRIN, STROKE, AND WOMEN

Like the aspirin–heart attack research, the aspirin-stroke studies focused primarily on men. Women comprised only one-quarter of the subjects in the six major trials.

Early on, it looked as though aspirin might not prevent stroke in women. In the 1978 Canadian Cooperative Study, aspirin reduced stroke risk in men 48 percent, but did not change it in women. That study, however, was one of the smaller trials—585 participants with only 179 women—raising the possibility of a Type II error. Every subsequent study—notably the two largest, which enrolled 2,500 participants with more than 600 women each—has shown no sex differences in aspirin benefits.

Most recently, a 1991 Finnish study with 2,500 participants with TIAs, 44 percent of whom were women, showed aspirin significantly beneficial for women as well as men. Compared with controls, after two years of daily treatment, 330 mg of aspirin (slightly more than one standard tablet) plus 75 mg of dipyridamole reduced stroke risk 49 percent in men and 41 percent in women. Although men benefited slightly more than women, the researchers wrote in the journal *Neurology,* "antiplatelet therapy is effective in the prevention of stroke in both sexes."

DOES ASPIRIN INCREASE RISK OF HEMORRHAGIC STROKE?

Based on the lower of the two meta-analysis results, aspirin prevents about 18 percent of ischemic strokes. Since about 80 percent of all strokes are ischemic, aspirin would appear to prevent 14.4 percent of total strokes (.80 × .18), or about 72,000 strokes each year. For a drug that costs less than a penny a day, this is miraculous.

But what about the other 20 percent of strokes that are hemorrhagic? Does aspirin's antiplatelet action, which prolongs bleeding, increase risk of cerebral and subarachnoid hemorrhage? It appeared to in the largest aspirin trial, the 22,000-participant Physicians' Health Study. Compared with the placebo group, the aspirin users suffered twice as many moderate-to-severe hemorrhagic strokes—thirteen versus six. Overall, stroke risk was tiny—less than 1 percent—and statistically insignificant. Nonetheless it was disturbing: "The possibility of an increase in hemorrhagic stroke among aspirin users," the researchers wrote, "is not unexpected, since any agent that decreases clotting may help prevent ischemic events, but increase bleeding."

As this book goes to press, aspirin's role, if any, in hemorrhagic stroke remains unclear. But anyone with stroke risk factors—particularly high blood pressure, bleeding problems, or a personal or family history of hemorrhagic stroke—should consult a physician before taking aspirin regularly.

ASPIRIN HELPS PREVENT SENILITY

Mention senility and most people think of Alzheimer's disease, the nation's leading cause of what doctors call "senile dementia." Alzheimer's slowly, inexorably destroys the minds of an estimated 10 percent of Americans aged 65 to 79 and up to 20 percent of those over 80. But Alzheimer's is not the only mind-robber. The nation's second leading cause of progressive mental deterioration is multi-infarct dementia (MID; "infarct" means "tissue death"). TIAs and ischemic strokes cause infarcts, or infarctions, in the brain, and multiple cerebral infarctions cause MID.

Neurologists are not sure what proportion of senile dementia is caused by MID. The estimates run from 15 to 47 percent. In addition, Alzheimer's disease and multi-infarct dementia can coexist. About one-fifth of those with senile dementia show signs of both.

Aspirin's success as a stroke preventive in those with TIAs and minor strokes spurred researchers to investigate whether its antithrombotic action might delay the progression of MID. A 1989 study at the Cerebral Blood Flow Laboratory at the Veterans Administration Medical Center in Houston showed that it not only slows the progression of MID but in some cases *reverses* it. Researchers divided seventy MID sufferers, average age 67, into two groups. One group received 325 mg of aspirin a day (one standard tablet), the other took no medication. The participants' cerebral blood flow and mental faculties were evaluated yearly. Some MID sufferers in both groups improved, some stabilized, and some deteriorated. Those taking aspirin stabilized or improved three-to-one over the controls. The aspirin group showed "significant improvement in cerebral [blood flow] and cognitive performance," the researchers concluded in the *Journal of the American Geriatrics Society*. "Their quality of life and independence appeared to improve. Daily aspirin appears to stabilize or improve cognition in multi-infarct dementia."

An accompanying editorial paid the study medicine's highest left-handed compliment. While calling the results "provocative" and "attractive to the clinician," it urged physicians not to start shoveling aspirin at everyone with MID until it had been corroborated. As this book goes to press, no corroborating study has been published, but many neurologists recommend daily low-dose aspirin treatment for those with MID.

NOT BY ASPIRIN ALONE

Aspirin's ability to prevent ischemic stroke is *no substitute* for reduction of the risk factors linked to atherosclerosis of the cerebral arteries. Control of high blood pressure is paramount. Aspirin reduces stroke risk about 18 percent, but a recent meta-analysis of fourteen studies involving 37,000 people showed that a six-point decrease in diastolic blood pressure (the second number in blood pressure readings) reduces stroke risk more than twice as much—42 percent. Nonsmokers have only half the stroke risk of smokers. The risk factors for stroke are the same as those for heart disease. See Chapter 1 for recommendations about controlling them.

Aspirin is the only over-the-counter drug known to reduce stroke risk, but several perscription drugs are more effective. Ticlopidine (Ticlid), approved in 1992, prevents ischemic stroke significantly better than aspirin, although its side effects may be considerably more severe. If you have a history of TIAs or minor strokes, consult your physician about appropriate drug therapy.

CHAPTER THREE

ASPIRIN HELPS PREVENT AND TREAT OTHER SERIOUS CARDIOVASCULAR CONDITIONS

PERIPHERAL ARTERY DISEASE

Atherosclerosis develops not only in the arteries that nourish the heart and brain but in other arteries as well, often those in the legs. The result is peripheral artery disease. When the leg arteries become narrowed beyond a certain point, intermittent claudication develops. Similar to angina (see Chapter 1), intermittent claudication causes leg pain, cramps, aching, or numbness. Symptoms typically appear during exercise and subside during rest. Sometimes the buttocks, hips, and thighs are affected, but symptoms usually develop in the calves, often accompanied by feelings of cold and numbness in the toes. Just as severe angina causes chest pain while at rest, those with serious intermittent claudication also experience symptoms while at rest. Possible other symptoms include: toenail thickening, leg swelling (edema), leg sores (ulcers), leg muscle atrophy, and gangrene (tissue death caused by loss of the local blood supply). Treatment sometimes requires amputation.

Men develop intermittent claudication more than women. The condition is strongly associated with smoking, high blood pressure, diabetes, and sedentary life-style. Quitting smoking, cholesterol and blood pressure control, and regular moderate exercise, particularly walking, swimming, and bicycling help relieve symptoms.

In severe cases, intermittent claudication may require bypass surgery, but most moderate cases are treatable with drugs, including aspirin. A 1990 study in the *Journal of Internal Medical Research* showed that aspirin combined with two other antiplatelet drugs (ticlopidine and dipyridamole) significantly improved blood flow and relieved symptoms.

According to a 1992 analysis of data from the Physicians' Health Study (see Chapter 1), aspirin alone helps prevent intermittent claudication. Compared with physicians in the control group, those who took one standard aspirin tablet every other day showed only half the risk. Among study participants who eventually required surgery for intermittent claudication, nine were from the control group, with only one from the aspirin group.

The small number of surgeries for severe intermittent claudication (only nine out of 22,000 study participants) made this risk reduction only barely statistically significant. But if this finding is confirmed by other research, it could have major implications. Each year 30,000 Americans have peripheral artery bypass surgery, and 37,000 endure an amputation because of severe peripheral artery disease. The researchers told *Family Practice News* that low-dose aspirin "could eliminate the need for a substantial number" of peripheral artery bypass operations.

DEEP VEIN THROMBOSIS

Veins, the blood vessels that return blood to the heart, are either superficial or deep. If a thrombus develops in a vein and causes inflammation, the condition is called "thrombophlebitis." Symptoms include swelling, warmth, redness, and pain. In a superficial vein, thrombophlebitis is painful but not life-threatening. However, if a thrombus in a deep vein travels into the lung (pulmonary embolism), death is a real possibility.

Each year about 300,000 Americans are hospitalized with deep vein thrombophlebitis, and this condition develops in up to 50 percent of those having surgical hip or knee replacements (arthroplasty). Deep vein thrombophlebitis is usually treated with anticoagulants, but a 1990 study at the University of North Carolina at Chapel Hill showed that aspirin helps prevent it.

Starting the night before their total hip replacements, 159 patients were given 650 mg of aspirin (two standard tablets). After surgery, they continued taking 650 mg of aspirin twice a day. Only 6 percent developed detectable deep vein thromboses. About 13 percent suffered pulmonary embolism but none died. Summarizing their pilot study in the *Journal of Arthroplasty,* the researchers suggested that aspirin looks promising as a way to prevent complications of hip replacement.

KIDNEY FAILURE:
VASCULAR ACCESS THROMBOSIS

The kidneys filter wastes, excess water, and chemicals out of the blood and turn them into urine. When the kidneys stop working (fail), wastes build up in the blood; without treatment this can eventually cause coma and death. Physicians treat advanced (end-stage) kidney failure in two ways: kidney transplants, and kidney machines, which cleanse the blood through hemodialysis (literally, taking the blood apart). Hemodialysis involves spending several hours two or three times a week hooked up to a kidney machine with blood from an arm or leg artery pumped through plastic tubing, filtered, and then returned to the body. Hemodialysis is a lifesaver, but sometimes thrombi develop in the arteries into which the tubing is plugged (vascular access thrombosis). According to a 1991 pilot study at the St. Louis School of Medicine in Missouri, aspirin helps prevent this condition. Researchers gave 85 mg of aspirin (one-quarter of a standard tablet) a day to fifteen hemodialysis patients with recurrent vascular access thrombosis. Writing in the journal *Thrombosis Research,* the researchers concluded that aspirin produces a "major reduction in frequency" of this complication.

CHAPTER FOUR

ASPIRIN MAY HELP
PREVENT COLON CANCER

Since the Physicians' Health Study results were published in 1988, medical excitement about aspirin has focused on its value in preventing heart attack and stroke, the nation's first and third leading causes of death. But in late 1991, aspirin suddenly appeared able to prevent the second leading cause of death as well—cancer, specifically colon cancer.

In a headline-making study in the *New England Journal of Medicine,* American Cancer Society (ACS) researchers showed that regular aspirin use reduced colon cancer deaths by 40 percent in men and 42 percent in women. This study has yet to be corroborated, and many questions about aspirin and colon cancer remain unanswered. Nonetheless, this study has persuaded many cancer specialists (oncologists) to jump on the aspirin bandwagon.

THE LEADING CANCER KILLER OF NONSMOKERS

Colon cancer is technically known as colorectal cancer, because it includes tumors of both the colon and rectum. Approximately 158,000 cases develop each year, one-third in the rectum, two-thirds in the colon. Colorectal cancer is the leading cause of cancer death after lung cancer, and the leading cancer killer of nonsmokers, claiming more than 58,000 lives each year. That's more than die annually from breast cancer (46,000), suicide (31,000), or homicide (21,000). Yet most people know little about this cancer because the area where it develops is considered unmentionable. When President Ronald Reagan developed the disease, the news media had a tough time discussing it. Today, many personal medical details, such as cholesterol levels, are subjects of everyday conversation, but colorectal cancer does not lend itself to casual chitchat.

Over the last twenty years, despite an enormous investment in early detection and treatment, the colorectal cancer death rate has declined only slightly. Yet early detection and treatment make a tremendous difference in survival. When colorectal tumors are detected and treated while still small and contained within the colorectal wall, the five-year survival rate (the proportion of people still alive five years after diagnosis) is better than 90 percent. If the disease is diagnosed after it has spread (metastasized), five-year survival is only about 10 percent. Unfortunately, highly publicized early-detection campaigns have had only modest success, and many cases are still diagnosed late, which makes the possibility of substantial death-rate reductions from regular aspirin use all the more exciting.

Colorectal cancer strikes men and women in equal numbers usually after age 50. In most cases, the tumors develop from slow-growing colonic nodules (polyps) that eventually turn cancerous. Early detection and surgical removal of these polyps is an important part of colorectal cancer prevention. The ACS recommends an internal examination (flexible sigmoidoscopy) at age 50 and every few years thereafter. Once colorectal tumors develop, they release tiny amounts of blood that become incorporated into the stool. This blood is invisible to the eye (occult) but detectable by a simple chemical test. The ACS recommends annual occult blood tests starting at age 50. Tragically, a 1989 ACS survey showed that only half of physicians recommend annual stool testing, and less than one-quarter follow ACS sigmoidoscopy recommendations.

Like cardiovascular disease, colorectal cancer has many risk factors, some controllable, some not. The ones that cannot be reduced include:

Age. The disease still usually develops after age 50, with peak incidence after 70. But in recent years it has increasingly been diagnosed in people in their 40s and even 30s.

Race. Colorectal cancer is slightly more prevalent among African Americans than among whites. (The National Cancer Institute [NCI] has not compiled data for other groups.)

Heredity. An estimated 20 percent of colorectal cancers have a genetic component. A rare but serious inherited condition called "familial polyposis of the colon" accounts for about 1 percent of colorectal cancers. Those with familial polyposis develop thousands of colon polyps in their 20s, some of which almost always turn cancerous by age 50. If you have any family history of colorectal cancer, ask your physician about the advisability of genetic counseling.

Even if you don't have familial polyposis, any colorectal cancer in a close relative—mother, father, sister, brother, grandparent, child, or blood-related aunt or uncle—increases your risk.

Colorectal cancer's controllable risk factors include: ·

Ulcerative colitis. In this disease, sores develop inside the colon, which cause abdominal pain, inflammation, and often bleeding. The longer the history of ulcerative colitis, the greater the risk of eventually developing colorectal cancer. Ulcerative colitis can often be treated with antiinflammatory medications. In severe cases, surgical removal of the colon may be necessary.

Asbestos exposure. Occupational exposure to asbestos fibers has been shown to increase risk of both lung and colorectal cancer.

Diet. For years, evidence has been accumulating that a diet high in fat and low in fiber increases risk. Colorectal cancer is very common in countries like the U.S. that have a high-fat, low-fiber diet—one heavy on red meats and light on fresh fruits and vegetables—but considerably less common in equally industrialized countries like Japan, whose residents eat a low-fat, high-fiber diet heavy on fruits, vegetables, and fish but light on red meats. The issue is still controversial because it remains unclear why dietary fat increases colorectal cancer risk, although most authorities believe that fat induces precancerous changes in the cells that line the colon. Nor is it clear why fresh fruits and vegetables provide protective benefits. For a while, scientists believed their fiber promoted the speedy passage of wastes through the colon, but now it appears that cancer-preventive chemicals in plant foods are equally, and perhaps more, important. Whatever the reasons, the diet-colorectal cancer link has been powerfully confirmed by three recent studies. A 1990 prospective investigation of the diets of 121,700 registered nurses in the *New England Journal of Medicine* showed that those who ate the most red meat had the highest colorectal cancer risk. Another 1990 report, a meta-analysis of many previous studies in the *Journal of the National Cancer Institute* showed that a diet high in fresh fruits and vegetables provided significant protection against the disease. Most recently, a 1992 evaluation of the diets of 7,000 American men also published in the *Journal of the National Cancer Institute* showed that a high-fat, low-fiber diet quadrupled the risk of colorectal polyps, the precursors of tumors.

FIFTEEN YEARS OF INTRIGUING DISCOVERIES

During the mid-1970s, as the first aspirin–heart attack trials were being published, cancer researchers reported that several kinds of animal and human tumors, including colorectal malignancies, produced elevated levels of prostaglandins, the same natural chemicals inhibited by aspirin, leading to the drug's prevention of heart attacks and ischemic strokes.

It didn't take long for scientists to test prostaglandin-inhibiting drugs on animal colorectal tumors to see if reducing their production of prostaglandins might slow the tumors' growth. Initially, two prostaglandin inhibitors were used, aspirin and indomethacin, one of many aspirinlike nonsteroidal antiinflammatory drugs (NSAIDs). A 1978 study published in the *British Journal of Cancer* showed that the drugs not only slowed animal colorectal tumor growth, but "in some cases, complete tumor elimination occurred."

Almost immediately, however, the prostaglandin-inhibition theory was challenged by other studies suggesting that indomethacin's antitumor effect was the result of immune system stimulation, which allowed cancer-stricken laboratory animals to fight the disease more successfully. The antiprostaglandin versus immune enhancement debate continues to this day.

From 1988 to 1991, four studies investigated the aspirin–colorectal cancer connection in humans. The first, by Australian researchers, examined the life-styles of 715 Melbourne colorectal cancer patients and 727 demographically similar healthy controls. Those with colorectal cancer had used significantly less aspirin and aspirin-containing drugs. Writing in the journal *Cancer Research,* the researchers concluded: "Aspirin . . . may be useful in the prevention of colorectal cancer."

Unfortunately, this study was retrospective. The researchers started with people with and without colorectal cancer and looked back in time to see if they could discern any life-style differences between them. Intriguing as these results were, retrospective studies are not as reliable as prospective trials that track people over time to see if the treatment being investigated has any effect. Nonetheless, the score was: one retrospective study pro, zero studies con.

The second trial, a 1989 study by University of Southern California researchers, was prospective, but unfortunately not placebo-controlled. It was based on a life-style questionnaire answered in 1981 by 13,987 residents of Leisure World, a retirement community near Los Angeles. The group was followed for more than six years using subsequent questionnaires and hospital records. Compared with those who did not use aspirin, those who took it daily showed 50 percent *more* colorectal cancers.

This finding was quite disturbing, but its impact was minimized by the study's other findings, which were also rather odd: The Leisure World population turned out to be "extraordinarily" healthy, the researchers wrote in the *British Medical Journal.* Based on actuarial tables, during the six-year study, 733 residents should have died, but remarkably, only 88 did. As a result, an unexpectedly small number of people developed colorectal cancer, casting doubt on any findings about the disease. In addition, the study showed that regular aspirin use also *increased risk of heart attack.* This finding, a year after publication of the Physicians' Health Study, raised a major red flag. Nonetheless, despite these problems, the Leisure World study was large and reasonably well-designed.

It made the score: one retrospective study pro, one prospective study con (but odd).

The third trial, a 1991 report by Boston University researchers, was a retrospective investigation comparing aspirin use among 1,326 people hospitalized with colorectal cancer and 4,891 controls, one-quarter of whom had other cancers. Regular aspirin use reduced the risk of colorectal cancer by about half, a statistically significant decrease. Those who took aspirin regularly for a while but who discontinued it more than a year before the study began showed no decrease in colorectal cancer risk, suggesting that any "protective effect is reversible after cessation," a finding that matched the results of earlier animal tests. Despite their retrospective study design, the researchers wrote in the *Journal of the National Cancer Institute:* "The regular use of NSAIDs reduces the incidence of human [colorectal] cancer." The score stood at: two retrospective studies pro, one prospective study con (but odd).

The balance was starting to tip in aspirin's favor against colorectal cancer, but before that could be firmly established, a prospective, double-blind, randomized, placebo-controlled trial had to be published. Later in 1991, one was, a French report in the journal *Gastroenterology.* Parisian researchers enrolled ten young adults, average age 37, who had familial polyposis, the inherited colorectal-polyp condition that almost always leads to cancer. Each received sulindac, an aspirinlike NSAID, for four months, and then a placebo for four months. (This is a "crossover" design. All subjects cross over from the treatment group to the placebo group.) While taking the NSAID, nine of the ten showed significant reductions in size and number of colorectal polyps. In six, polyps disappeared. But when they switched to the placebo, their polyps returned and grew. Despite the small number of subjects, the results were statistically significant. Of course, sulindac is not aspirin, but this study lent additional credence to NSAIDs', including aspirin's, effectiveness against colorectal cancer. The score was now: three studies pro, one con (but odd).

The balance tipped even further in aspirin's favor with the late 1991 publication of the American Cancer Society study mentioned at the beginning of this chapter. In this large prospective trial, researchers reexamined diet and life-style questionnaires, including information on aspirin consumption, completed by more than 600,000 Americans in the early 1980s. Six years later, the regular aspirin users had a death rate from colorectal cancer 40 percent lower than the controls. Those who took the drug at least sixteen times a month suffered the fewest deaths. The score stood at: four studies pro, one con (but odd).

The enormous size of the ACS study lent credence to its conclusions, but its reliance on a drug-recall survey detracted from it. In addition, it focused only on death from colorectal cancer, not on diagnosis of the disease. An editorial accompanying the study called the findings "intriguing" but far from conclusive. While it may not have been the colorectal version of the Physicians' Health Study, its impressive findings and its publication in the nation's leading medical journal sent millions of cancer-phobic Americans rushing to their medicine cabinets.

THE BIG QUESTION: WHY?

As this book goes to press, aspirin looks promising—very promising—against colorectal cancer, but the case for its regular use is nowhere near as strong as the case for aspirin prevention of heart attack and stroke. Even if subsequent studies confirm the ACS trial, many physicians may remain reluctant to recommend it for this purpose if only because no one is sure why it works (if it really does). Theories abound.

Aspirin might fight colorectal cancer by blocking tumor production of growth-promoting prostaglandins. It may also boost the immune system's ability to fight this cancer. Animal data suggest both possibilities, and the human research, particularly the familial polyposis study, might be explained either way.

Then there's the possibility that the aspirin's value against colorectal cancer might hinge on one of its well-known side effects—promotion of gastrointestinal bleeding. As colon tumors develop, they release tiny amounts of blood detectable in the stool using the occult blood test the ACS recommends annually for everyone over 50. Those taking occult blood tests are not supposed to take aspirin for several days beforehand because aspirin-related gastrointestinal bleeding might produce a false-positive test result. But let's suppose that aspirin spurs tumor bleeding for a few weeks. If people stopped using the drug several days before occult blood tests, their tumors might still be more likely to bleed and produce a positive result, leading to additional tests that might diagnose early-stage tumors and allow unusually early treatment and better survival. It's also possible that significant numbers of regular aspirin users might forget or ignore the no-aspirin admonition, and have false-positive occult blood tests, leading to additional tests and diagnosis of tumors too small to turn the test positive by themselves. No one knows. Until aspirin's mechanism of action has been determined, its role (if any) in colorectal cancer prevention will remain an open question.

NOT BY ASPIRIN ALONE

Even if aspirin is effective against colorectal cancer, the drug is *no substitute* for reduction of the risk factors linked to this disease.

• If any close relative has had colorectal cancer, mention
it to your physician and consider colorectal cancer screening
more frequently and starting at an earlier age than the ACS
recommends. If any relative developed the disease before age
50, you may have familial polyposis. Ask your physician for
an examination.

• Have an occult blood test annually after age 50.

• Have a sigmoidoscopy at age 50 and every three years
after that. One recent study showed that regular sigmoidoscopy reduces deaths from colorectal cancer by 59 percent.

• Eat a low-fat diet based on whole grains and fresh fruits
and vegetables. See *Eater's Choice* by Ron and Nancy Goor
(Resources).

CHAPTER FIVE

ASPIRIN AND PREGNANCY: SIGNIFICANT RISKS, MAJOR NEW BENEFITS

Aspirin was once the expectant mother's friend. Millions of women took it as their home remedy for the discomforts of pregnancy. But over the last thirty years, many animal and human studies have linked aspirin to an increased risk of several pregnancy complications, including birth defects. As a result, by the late 1970s, the drug was vilified as the pregnant woman's enemy. Aspirin's role in human defects remains controversial; nonetheless, most physicians discourage therapeutic doses (two tablets every four hours) during pregnancy, particularly during the last three months (third trimester) of pregnancy, because the drug is associated with excessive bleeding during delivery.

On the other hand, the latest research has transformed *low-dose* aspirin back into the friend—often the savior—of the 10 percent of women who develop pregnancy-induced hypertension (PIH), a sudden increase in maternal blood pressure that can cause convulsions in expectant mothers and serious problems, even death, in their babies. Sixty to 150 mg of aspirin a day have been shown to prevent PIH and one other serious complication of pregnancy.

COMPLICATIONS AND POSSIBLY BIRTH DEFECTS

Until 1960, physicians thought few medications crossed the placenta from mother to unborn child. As a result, common drugs, particularly over-the-counter products like aspirin, were considered safe during pregnancy until proven otherwise. Then came thalidomide, a supposedly safe over-the-counter sedative taken by tens of thousands of pregnant European women that caused more than 8,000 of their children to be born with seal-like flippers instead of arms and legs. The thalidomide scandal hit the headlines just as the Food and Drug Administration (FDA) was preparing to approve the drug for marketing in the U.S. Approval was quickly denied. The FDA began insisting on more thorough manufacturer safety tests of new drugs, regulations still largely in place today. The pendulum on drug use during pregnancy began swinging to the current view that all drugs, including over-the-counter products, are hazardous to the fetus until proven otherwise.

Unfortunately, the message has had a tough time getting through. Twelve years ago, a study of 50,000 American women showed that 64 percent used aspirin at some point during pregnancy, and that 30 percent took it during the first trimester, when drugs are most likely to cause serious fetal damage. Since then, major educational efforts have discouraged drug use during pregnancy, but they have been only modestly effective. In a 1987 study of 500 pregnant women, 46 percent reported taking aspirin at least once, making it one of the three most widely used drugs during pregnancy (along with caffeine and acetaminophen).

It's a mistake to take therapeutic doses of aspirin (two tablets every four hours) during pregnancy unless your doctor recommends it. Many studies show that it can harm both mother and child.

Maternal bleeding. Compared with pregnant women who take no aspirin, those who consume three to five standard tablets a day within ten days of delivery lose about 40 percent more blood while giving birth. Aspirin use earlier in pregnancy does not increase delivery-related blood loss, nor do low doses of up to 150 mg a day taken at any time. Excess blood loss does increase medical risks, and given the uncertainty of time of delivery, most physicians discourage aspirin during the entire third trimester of normal pregnancies.

Newborn bleeding. Studies of laboratory animals and full-term human infants show that fetal exposure to aspirin increases bleeding problems in newborns. This discovery led to studies of prenatal aspirin exposure's effect on premature, very-low-birth-weight infants, about one-third of whom suffer bleeding inside the head (intracranial hemorrhage). In one study among pregnant women who took one to five aspirin tablets during the week before delivery, their premature newborns suffered intracranial hemorrhage at more than double the expected rate. About 9 percent of U.S. infants are born prematurely, and approximately 1 percent—40,000 babies a year—are classified as having very low birth weight. If aspirin doubles risk of intracranial hemorrhage, the drug might be responsible for thousands of cases a year. This is another reason why physicians discourage aspirin during the last trimester. (Prenatal acetaminophen exposure is not associated with intracranial hemorrhage.)

Prolonged gestation. In cases of threatened premature labor, physicians try to prolong gestation. But past term, additional gestation can become a problem. Prostaglandins play a role in uterine contractions and the opening of the cervix shortly before delivery. Because aspirin interferes with prostaglandin action, scientists theorized that it might also prolong gestation. Several animal studies have shown this to be true, and two studies of rheumatoid arthritis sufferers, who took aspirin regularly during pregnancy, showed that their babies arrived about a week later than average. Put another way, the normal risk of having a postmature delivery is 4 percent; among regular aspirin users it's 16 percent.

Prolonged labor. No one wants a long labor. One study detected no differences in the labor of regular aspirin users and nonusers. But another showed that compared with normal women, who labored an average of seven hours, those with rheumatoid arthritis labored 12 hours—70 percent longer. None of the normal women labored longer than 24 hours, but 17 percent of the arthritis group did. Prolonged labor is another reason pregnant women should steer clear of the pain reliever doctors recommend most. (Low-dose aspirin use during pregnancy does not prolong labor.)

Birth defects. Aspirin was first shown to cause birth defects in the pups of pregnant rats way back in 1959. Since then, many studies have confirmed the effect and extended it to cats, dogs, and monkeys. Most aspirin-related birth defects are heart malformations. Epidemiologists now consider aspirin a "definitive" cause of birth defects in animals. The drug's effect in humans is considerably less clear—the studies go both ways. Some show no increased risk of birth defects in the children of women who used aspirin during pregnancy. Others, particularly studies of aspirin use during the first trimester, show unexpectedly large numbers of children born with heart problems, cleft palates, and abnormal hands and feet. Reviewers have questioned the quality of the studies showing aspirin-related birth defects. But better safe than sorry. Pregnant women should not take aspirin unless advised to do so by a physician.

LOW-DOSE ASPIRIN: PREVENTION OF PREGNANCY-INDUCED HYPERTENSION

After the twentieth week of pregnancy, about 10 percent of women develop high blood pressure, a condition once known as toxemia of pregnancy, but now called "pregnancy-induced hypertension" (PIH). PIH has three levels of severity. In some women, elevated blood pressure is the only symptom. In others, fluid retention (edema) and/or protein in the urine (proteinuria) occur along with hypertension, resulting in pre-eclampsia, which significantly increases risk of maternal death and fetal growth retardation and death. In severe cases, PIH triggers convulsions (eclampsia), which causes even higher rates of maternal and fetal death.

An estimated 20 percent of pregnancy-related maternal deaths are caused by PIH, and as recently as 1989, a popular obstetrics textbook called the condition "among the most important unsolved problems in obstetrics." Recently, the mystery was solved, and today, low-dose aspirin is saving thousands of maternal and fetal lives.

Any woman can develop PIH, but there are risk factors:

First pregnancies. About two-thirds of women who develop PIH have carried no other pregnancy to term.

Age. Compared with women in their 20s, pregnant women over 40 have three times the risk of PIH—10 percent as opposed to 3 percent.

Race. White women have the lowest risk of PIH. Hispanic women develop it somewhat more frequently. African-American women are at highest risk.

Heredity. Daughters of women who had PIH are at increased risk.

Obstetricians and many others have speculated on the cause of PIH for decades. "Everyone from allergist to zoologist has proposed a theory," according to F. Gary Cunningham, M.D., chair of the Department of Obstetrics and Gynecology at the University of Texas's Southwestern Medical Center. But none of the suggested mechanisms led to an effective treatment, so one by one, the theories were discarded.

However, back in 1979, Italian researchers published a little-noticed report in *The Lancet* on a curious aspect of aspirin's action on blood clotting. As discussed in Chapter 1, when blood vessels rupture and bleed, the cells at the injury site release arachidonic acid. The enzyme cyclooxygenase transforms it into the prostaglandin thromboxane-A_2, which triggers platelet aggregation and clotting. Aspirin interferes with the action of cyclooxygenase and inhibits the formation of thromboxane, which is the basis for its effectiveness against heart attack, ischemic stroke, and other thrombotic conditions. But thromboxane is not the only prostaglandin produced when arachidonic acid comes in contact with cyclooxygenase. Another product of their union is prostacyclin. Intuitively, one might expect that aspirin's interference with cyclooxygenase would inhibit the formation of both thromboxane and prostacyclin. The Italian researchers showed, however, that while aspirin stops thromboxane synthesis completely, it depresses prostacyclin only slightly.

During the early 1980s, studies showed that thromboxane does more than just trigger platelet aggregation. It also narrows the blood vessels (vasoconstriction). Prostacyclin, on the other hand, widens them (vasodilation). Vasoconstrictors raise blood pressure because the heart has to pump harder to push blood through narrower blood vessels. Vasodilators reduce blood pressure because blood circulates more easily through open blood vessels and the heart doesn't have to work as hard.

Thromboxane's and prostacyclin's effects on blood vessels were not connected to PIH until 1985 when Scott Walsh of

Michigan State turned up something unexpected about women who developed the condition. In normal pregnancies, levels of both thromboxane and prostacyclin rise together. But in women with PIH, the rise in thromboxane is not matched by an increase in prostacyclin. Walsh speculated in the *American Journal of Obstetrics and Gynecology* that this discrepancy might explain PIH. An unusually low level of vasodilating prostacyclin would not offset the relative excess of vasoconstricting thromboxane, and the net effect would narrow the blood vessels and increase blood pressure. If Walsh were right, then a selective thromboxane inhibitor that did not decrease prostacyclin might restore the normal ratio of the two prostaglandins and prevent PIH. There was only one— aspirin.

By the time this study was published, it was clear from the aspirin–heart disease work that very low doses inhibited thromboxane. Given the potentially fatal consequences of PIH, aspirin seemed worth a try, even at the risk of causing some of the problems discussed earlier in this chapter.

From 1985 to 1990, six small clinical trials investigated daily low-dose aspirin's effects on second- and third-trimester women at risk for PIH:

- A 1985 study of 102 women by French researchers showed no cases of PIH in the half treated with 150 mg of aspirin, but 6 among the untreated controls.
- A 1986 report on 46 women by Dutch investigators showed 2 cases of mild PIH in the half treated with 60 mg of aspirin, but 12 cases, including one case of convulsions, in those who did not take the drug.
- A 1987 study of 48 pregnancies by the same Dutch researchers showed 2 cases of mild PIH in the half taking about 75 mg of aspirin, but 4 cases in the controls.
- A 1989 report on 33 women by Italian researchers showed no cases of PIH in the half taking 60 mg of aspirin, but 3 among the untreated controls.

• Another 1989 study of 65 pregnancies by Israeli researchers showed 4 cases of PIH in the half treated with 100 mg of aspirin, versus 11 cases among the controls.

• Finally, a 1990 report on 100 women by British researchers showed 6 cases of PIH in the half given 75 mg of aspirin, but 13 cases among the untreated controls.

Five of the six PIH results were statistically significant. In addition, all six showed no significant increase in bleeding problems among the women or the babies exposed to aspirin. And all six showed that the aspirin-exposed newborns had longer gestations (meaning less risk of medically hazardous prematurity) and greater birth weights (meaning less risk of hazardous low birth weight).

Unfortunately, all six clinical trials involved relatively small numbers of women, raising suspicions of experimental error. A 1991 meta-analysis in *The Journal of the American Medical Association* laid that possibility soundly to rest. Case Western Reserve researchers combined the six results and showed that aspirin treatment reduced risk of PIH by 65 percent, and risk of very low birth weight by 44 percent. In addition, the Case Western researchers pointed out that women with PIH often must deliver by cesarean section, which is medically riskier and much more costly than vaginal birth. By minimizing risk of PIH, aspirin treatment also reduced C-sections by 66 percent. "Low-dose aspirin," the Case Western team wrote, "is a highly efficacious and safe preventive therapy for PIH and its [complications]."

LOW-DOSE ASPIRIN: TWO MORE BENEFITS

Aspirin has also been used successfully to treat two other serious complications of pregnancy—umbilical placental insufficiency (UPI) and lupus anticoagulant abortion.

The placenta is the organ inside the womb that connects the fetus with the mother. It takes food and oxygen from the maternal blood supply and sends it via the umbilical cord to the fetus. It also takes fetal wastes and returns them to the mother for elimination. The placenta develops as the fetus grows and is expelled shortly after delivery. In umbilical placental insufficiency, the placenta does not function properly, and the fetus becomes undernourished, resulting in fetal growth retardation with low birth weight and, in severe cases, fetal death. Scientists are still not sure what causes UPI, but presumably a thromboxane-prostacyclin imbalance plays a key role because several studies have shown that low-dose aspirin treatment produces a "drastic reduction" in mild to moderate fetal growth retardation, and "significantly improved" pregnancy outcomes.

CHAPTER SIX

THE NEW ASPIRIN FRONTIER

In the future, aspirin may be used for more than the prevention of heart attack, angina, stroke, multi-infarct dementia, other cardiovascular conditions, colorectal cancer, and pregnancy-induced hypertension. Scientists are currently investigating several other intriguing possibilities.

The findings summarized in this chapter are preliminary. If you have any of the conditions mentioned, alert your physician to the possibility that aspirin might help—many physicians are unaware of this research—and point out the appropriate journal citations in the References for this chapter, located at the back of this book. Don't take aspirin regularly without your physician's approval, but assuming that you have no health problems precluding its use, your physician might advise you to try it.

ASPIRIN MAY HELP
PREVENT MIGRAINE HEADACHES

The British Doctors' Study and the U.S. Physicians' Health Study, both discussed in Chapter 1, did more than prove that low-dose aspirin prevents heart attacks in healthy men. They also linked regular aspirin use to migraine headache prevention.

Compared with heart attack, migraines are medically minor, yet the searingly painful headaches are a major affliction for more than 25 million women and 8 million men in the United States. Migraines cause several hours to two days of severe, sometimes disabling, throbbing head pain, usually on one side, often accompanied by nausea and vomiting.

Researchers are uncertain what causes migraines, but before they strike, the small arteries in the brain (arterioles) become constricted, reducing cerebral blood flow. Migraines are not classically hereditary, but they often run in families. More than 60 percent of migraine sufferers have a family history of severe headaches. Sometimes migraines have specific triggers: exercise, emotional stress, exposure to intense sunlight, birth control pills, premenstrual fluid retention, alcohol (particularly red wine), milk and wheat products, and caffeine (coffee, tea, chocolate, colas, and some over-the-counter drugs, for example the aspirin-caffeine combination in Anacin and the aspirin-acetaminophen-caffeine combination in Excedrin).

In 1977, researchers discovered that changes in platelet aggregation seemed to be involved in migraine attacks, and the following year, a placebo-controlled trial in *The Lancet* showed that regular aspirin consumption reduced migraine frequency by 50 percent. But that result was based on only twelve subjects, too few to gain much attention.

During the 1980s, migraine researchers generally focused their preventive efforts on relaxing constricted arterioles by prescribing more than twenty different drugs, particularly blood pressure medications, and the platelet work lost its allure.

It was persuasively resurrected in 1988 by the two doctor studies. Both were large clinical trials, and both used state-of-the-art, prospective, randomized, double-blind, placebo-controlled designs. In the British study, the aspirin users reported 30 percent fewer migraines. In the American study, the figure was 20 percent.

Presumably, in these two studies, aspirin's antiplatelet effect was responsible for the reductions in migraines, but at this writing, many questions remain unanswered. Nonetheless, writing in the *Journal of the American Medical Association,* the researchers who evaluated the American data concluded that "migraine is [triggered], at least in part, by the effects of platelets." Aspirin "should be considered" for migraine prevention.

Other studies have shown that beta-blockers, a type of blood pressure medication, prevent migraines better than aspirin. But no single migraine-preventive drug works for everyone. Aspirin may not be your physician's first-choice drug for migraine prevention, but it should be on the list.

ASPIRIN MAY HELP PREVENT CATARACTS

Cataracts are cloudy, opaque areas that develop in the eye's normally clear lens. Cataracts block or distort light entering the eye, and over time impair vision. As cataracts develop, they interfere with color perception, making the world look increasingly gray. During the day, objects appear increasingly indistinct, as though veiled behind gauze. At night, driving becomes difficult, then impossible, because objects disappear in the glare of oncoming headlights. If untreated, cataracts can cause blindness. Cataracts are not related to eyestrain; they usually develop slowly over several years but may advance rapidly in just a few months.

There are several kinds of cataracts, but three-quarters are associated with aging (senile cataracts). The cloudy areas usually develop in both eyes, but typically one is more affected than the other. Other risk factors include: smoking, diabetes, nearsightedness (myopia), a family history, certain eye injuries, corticosteroid drug use, and exposure to radiation.

If vision loss becomes serious, the clouded lens can be removed surgically and replaced with an artificial lens, or the person can be fitted with special glasses or contact lenses. About 1 million Americans have cataract surgery each year at an estimated cost of $2.5 billion.

Until the late 1970s, physicians believed that senile cataracts could not be prevented. But in 1991 the same epidemiological analysis that identified smoking and exposure to radiation as important cataracts risk factors pointed to preventive value for quitting smoking and wearing eye protection. It also showed decreased risk for those with diets high in vitamins A, C, E, riboflavin, niacin, thiamine, and iron, and those who take a multivitamin supplement at least once a week. Over the last decade, evidence has accumulated that aspirin also helps prevent cataracts.

The aspirin-cataracts story began in 1981 when two studies independently documented a surprisingly low incidence of cataracts in people with rheumatoid arthritis, who typically take large doses of aspirin throughout their lives. If aspirin does help prevent cataracts, the mechanism remains unclear. Presumably, aspirin somehow interferes with the chemical changes that cloud the lens.

Only a handful of studies have pursued the aspirin-cataract question. The results have been inconclusive:

• A 1982 report involving 2,675 participants in the Framingham Eye Study, an offshoot of the better-known Framingham Heart Study, showed no cataract-preventive value for aspirin. However, its publication in the journal *Ophthal-*

mology was followed by a critique dismissing it as "invalid" for allegedly poor methodology.

• A 1989 study of twelve cataract sufferers published by Indian researchers showed that compared with controls, one standard aspirin tablet taken three times a day significantly slowed cataract development. But this study's small subject pool raises questions about its findings.

• A 1989 study of 1,031 cataract patients by British researchers showed that regular aspirin (and ibuprofen) use "was associated with a halving of risk of cataract development."

• But a 1991 report based on the 22,071 participants in the Physicians' Health Study proved disappointing. Physicians in the aspirin group developed somewhat fewer cataracts and had 20 percent fewer cataract operations than controls, but the differences were statistically insignificant. Nonetheless, the researchers "could not exclude a small to moderate benefit of alternate-day, low-dose aspirin."

Given the prevalence of cataracts and the frequency and cost of cataract surgery, the aspirin-cataract issue deserves more study. If you have cataracts or are at risk, ask your physician about the advisability of taking aspirin. If it does you no harm, it might do you some good.

ASPIRIN MAY HELP PREVENT GALLSTONES

Gallstones are solid pellets that form in the gallbladder, which is located in the upper right portion of the abdomen under the rib cage. Some cause severe pain, which typically starts a half hour after eating, builds to an intense peak, then subsides after an hour or so. Fever and vomiting are also possible.

About 20 million Americans—mostly women—have gallstones, and a million new cases are diagnosed yearly. Until recently, more than 300,000 Americans had gallbladder surgery each year to remove gallstones, and about 6,000 died from surgical complications. Now new stone-dissolving drugs and nonsurgical shock-wave treatments (lithotripsy) are becoming more popular; still, gallbladder surgery continues to be performed. Fortunately, most gallstones can be prevented.

The gallbladder stores bile, a liver secretion that helps the body digest fats. Bile is a mixture of many substances but the one most likely to form gallstones is cholesterol, which accounts for about 75 percent of all cases of stones. The cholesterol concentration of bile increases in the presence of estrogen, the female sex hormone, which is why women develop gallstones more often than men. Anything that increases a woman's estrogen level—pregnancy, birth control pills, or postmenopausal estrogen replacement therapy—increases her risk of gallstones.

Other risk factors include: smoking, diabetes, obesity, high blood pressure, and a high-fat diet, which increases cholesterol. Controlling these risk factors helps prevent gallstones. Aspirin might, too—animal studies in the early 1980s showed that aspirin treatment helped prevent gallstones.

In 1988, European researchers surveyed gallstone sufferers and discovered that regular use of nonsteroidal antiinflammatory drugs (NSAIDs) significantly decreased the likelihood of recurrences. Of the twelve regular NSAID users, five took aspirin in daily doses ranging from 400 to 1,200 mg (approximately one to four standard tablets).

However, two UCLA studies have been disappointing. In a 1988 report researchers showed that aspirin (1,300 mg a day, or four standard tablets) prevented pregallstone chemical changes in bile but did not decrease the number of stones formed. And a large 1991 reanalysis of the 4,524 participants in the AMIS study (see Chapter 1) showed that compared with controls, those who took a daily dose of 1,000 mg of aspirin (about three standard tablets) were just as likely to have been hospitalized for gallstones, suggesting no protective effect for aspirin.

As this book goes to press, aspirin cannot be considered effective in preventing gallstones. But it has not been shown to be completely ineffective either. If you have had gallstones, or if you're at risk, ask your physician about the advisability of taking aspirin.

ASPIRIN MAY HELP PREVENT DIABETIC EYE PROBLEMS

An estimated 12 million Americans have diabetes, and the disease is a factor in more than 250,000 deaths each year, making it one of the nation's most serious medical problems. Diabetes occurs when the body stops producing the pancreatic hormone insulin, or becomes unable to use the insulin it produces. Without insulin, blood sugar (glucose), the body's major fuel, cannot be used by the cells. It builds up in the bloodstream and eventually turns up in the urine. The high sugar content of the urine draws water out of the body, causing increased urination and thirst. Diabetes also changes the way the body processes fats, increasing the risk of atherosclerosis and, as a result, heart disease and stroke. In addition, diabetes narrows the body's small blood vessels, impairing circulation, which may interfere with wound healing and cause kidney disease and foot and eye problems (retinopathy).

In diabetic retinopathy, some of the blood vessels in the eye's nerve-rich retina die while others leak blood, impairing vision. Control of blood sugar, either through diet or by injecting insulin, helps prevent retinopathy, and if the condition is detected early, laser surgery may be able to control it. Nonetheless, fifteen years after diagnosis, two-thirds of diabetics show signs of eye damage, and each year diabetic retinopathy causes blindness in about 5,000 Americans.

Most diabetics die of cardiovascular disease, so diabetologists followed the aspirin–heart attack and aspirin-stroke research closely. As the case for aspirin's preventive value grew stronger, they began recommending it to diabetics. But there was a catch. Many physicians feared that regular aspirin use by diabetics might involve a disturbing trade-off: less risk of heart attack and stroke but possibly *increased* risk of blindness if aspirin's antiplatelet effect caused more bleeding in the eye. Fortunately, diabetics who took aspirin to prevent cardiovascular disease did not show significantly greater risk of retinopathy. In fact, studies in the early 1980s suggested that retinopathy seemed linked to abnormally sticky platelets, raising the hope that aspirin might help prevent *both* cardiovascular disease and diabetic eye problems.

As this book goes to press, two aspirin-retinopathy studies have been published—with mixed results:

• A 1989 trial by British and French researchers involving 475 diabetics with early retinopathy showed that compared with controls, those who took 330 mg of aspirin (about one standard tablet) three times a day for three years showed significantly less eye deterioration.

• But aspirin showed no protective benefit in a ten-year study published in 1991 by U.S. National Eye Institute researchers who studied 3,711 diabetics with retinopathy. Compared with the placebo group, those who took a daily dose of 650 mg of aspirin (two standard tablets) experienced just as much progressive vision impairment.

Compared with the European study, the larger size and longer duration of the National Eye Institute trial gives it greater scientific weight. But the question of aspirin's effect, if any, on diabetic retinopathy remains open. If you have diabetes, ask your physician about the advisability of taking aspirin.

ASPIRIN HAS CONFUSING
EFFECTS ON THE IMMUNE SYSTEM

Until the early 1980s, when AIDS emerged as a serious world health problem, few nonphysicians knew much about the immune system, the complex collection of white blood cells, antibodies, and dozens of other proteins that defend the body against disease. Destruction of the immune system by the AIDS virus has spurred tremendous interest in the body's defensive system—and in anything that enhances it. During the mid-1970s, it looked as if aspirin suppressed the immune system; by the late 1980s, research suggested that aspirin stimulated it and had an antiviral effect. The latest study, however, again suggests immune suppression.

Back in 1975, a study of aspirin's effects on the common cold by University of Illinois researchers showed that compared with cold sufferers who took no aspirin, those who did released (shed) more virus and were, presumably, more likely to spread their colds. The researchers concluded that aspirin use by cold sufferers might be an "epidemiological hazard."

Why would aspirin increase viral shedding? Initially, researchers focused on aspirin's well-known fever-reducing (antipyretic) effect. Few adults develop noticeable fevers from colds, but body temperature does rise somewhat. The increase helps fight the infection. Cold viruses—and many other disease organisms—have difficulty reproducing at temperatures much above normal body temperature. It seemed reasonable to believe that by lowering body temperature, aspirin might contribute to increased viral reproduction and shedding.

Aspirin's antipyretic effect was only part of the story. During the 1980s, a few pilot studies suggested that aspirin suppressed production of interferon, the immune system's antiviral chemical. A few years later, more sophisticated studies persuasively showed the opposite. Aspirin actually *stimulates* production of interferon and interleukin-2, another important immune system protein.

In 1988, George Washington University researchers gave twenty young adults either a placebo or one standard aspirin tablet every other day for six days. After the first dose, the subjects were infected with colds. The aspirin group produced two to five times as much interferon and interleukin-2. Another study by researchers at the University of California at Irvine confirmed aspirin's ability to stimulate interferon production.

That same year, in a test-tube study, German researchers reported that aspirin inhibits influenza (flu) virus, suggesting an antiviral effect.

But in 1991, Australian researchers showed that aspirin and acetaminophen (Tylenol, Anacin-3, etc.) both suppress antibody production, another component of the immune system.

These conflicting reports add up to a puzzle. Aspirin may increase viral shedding, but no studies have shown that it contributes to spreading colds. Aspirin may stimulate production of interferon and interleukin-2, but no studies have shown that it shortens colds. Aspirin may suppress antibody production, but no studies have shown that it lengthens colds. The only real-world effect discovered so far has been the recent Australian finding that compared with cold sufferers who take ibuprofen (Advil, Nuprin, Motrin, etc.), those who use aspirin or acetaminophen suffer more runny nose and nasal congestion. Aspirin's effects on the overall functioning of the immune system remain a mystery.

ASPIRIN MAY HELP PREVENT INSOMNIA

Insomnia is one of the nation's leading medical complaints. One-third to one-half of the population has trouble falling or staying asleep at some time in life, and some 10 million Americans suffer chronic insomnia.

During the 1960s and early 1970s, a half-dozen studies suggested that aspirin has a mild sedative effect in animals and humans. In 1980, the director of the Dartmouth Sleep Clinic in New Hampshire compared placebo and aspirin treatment (two standard tablets before bed) in chronic insomniacs. After three weeks, the aspirin group showed significant benefit. Unfortunately, this study was small, just eight subjects, so its results don't carry much weight.

Aspirinlike salicylates are included in some over-the-counter sleep aids on the theory that pain is a frequent cause of insomnia. If so, aspirin's pain-relieving action should help people *fall* asleep, but when the drug wears off, pain might be expected to return, so aspirin should be less likely to help people *stay* asleep. Curiously, in the Dartmouth study, aspirin had no effect on the time it took subjects to fall asleep; it did help them stay asleep during the second half of the night. As this book goes to press, this study has not been followed up. It should be.

Unlike other sleep aids, aspirin causes no morning grogginess; unlike prescription sleeping pills, aspirin is nonaddictive. The Dartmouth researchers concluded: "It would seem prudent to use aspirin as a first line of defense against occasional insomnia." If you'd like to try it, consult your physician.

ASPIRIN MAY HELP
OBESE WOMEN LOSE WEIGHT

Most people use the term *obese* in a general way to mean "fat." Medically, it has a more precise definition: 20 percent over the recommended weight for your height and build.

For most people, weight control involves a combination of a low-fat, low-alcohol diet and regular moderate exercise. Those who are seriously obese often need professional help.

One contributor to some people's obesity is a low basal metabolic rate (BMR), the body's rate of calorie consumption when resting. The higher your BMR, the more calories you burn throughout the day, and the more you can consume without gaining weight. Exercise not only burns calories, it also raises BMR, which means that physical activity contributes to weight control even when you're not exercising.

Since the mid-1980s, obesity researchers have been experimenting with drugs that raise BMR, particularly ephedrine, a noncaffeine stimulant chemically related to pseudoephedrine, the decongestant in many over-the-counter cold and allergy formulas such as Sudafed. Several studies have shown that obese women lose more weight when enrolled in medically supervised weight-loss programs that include ephedrine treatment. One 1991 study by British researchers in the *International Journal of Obesity* shows that compared with ephedrine by itself, ephedrine plus 300 mg of aspirin (slightly less than one standard tablet) raises BMR significantly more.

Curiously, ephedrine and ephedrine-plus-aspirin raise BMR *only* in medically obese women, not those of average weight or those slightly overweight. If you want to lose five or ten pounds, you won't get much help from aspirin, but if you're clinically obese and would like to give your BMR an extra boost, mention this study to your physician.

ASPIRIN MAY HELP PREVENT
WHEAT INTOLERANCE

Difficulty digesting wheat, specifically the wheat protein gluten, affects an estimated several million Americans. Physicians call the condition gluten intolerance or gluten enteropathy. Symptoms include chronic abdominal distress and diarrhea. Once diagnosed, physicians typically recommend avoiding foods that contain gluten. That's easier said than done—gluten is almost everywhere.

In 1982, a Texas researcher who suffered from gluten intolerance wrote *The Lancet* about an experiment he performed on himself:

> Increased prostaglandin levels have been found in the stool of patients with several gastrointestinal diseases. Because aspirin inhibits prostaglandin [synthesis, a recent study published in this journal has shown aspirin] effective for preventing the symptoms of some food-intolerant gastrointestinal diseases. As a sufferer from gluten intolerance, I have been experimenting with aspirin.
>
> [After my diagnosis], a gluten-free diet provided relief of all my symptoms. But whenever I ate gluten inadvertently, my symptoms returned immediately. After I had been on the gluten-free diet for a year, I challenged [myself] with gluten-containing foods after aspirin treatment. Taking 650 mg five to 15 minutes before a meal completely prevented all symptoms of gluten enteropathy, irrespective of how much gluten the meal contained. Taking aspirin after the meal was not protective. I have taken aspirin before gluten-containing meals for a year. It has never failed to prevent gluten enteropathy symptoms. I know of one other person with adult-onset gluten enteropathy who has also successfully used aspirin to prevent acute symptoms.

Case reports like this one are intriguing, but they cannot be considered scientifically persuasive. As this book goes to press, no clinical trials have been published. But if you have gluten intolerance, mention this report to your physician. If aspirin does you no harm, it might help you return to eating pizza.

ASPIRIN MAY PREVENT HIP
REPLACEMENT COMPLICATIONS

Each year, more than 135,000 Americans have hip replacements (total hip arthroplasty) for joint destruction caused by arthritis or osteoporosis (bone-thinning due to calcium loss, a particular problem in postmenopausal women).

About half of those who have hip replacements develop a complication called "heterotopic ossification," or bony growths around the artificial joint. In approximately 10,000 hip-replacement patients per year, this complication causes chronic pain and restricts the new joint's range of motion. Sometimes the replacement joint becomes useless.

Since 1988, several studies have shown that the aspirinlike drug indomethacin prevents heterotopic ossification, but side effects preclude its use in more than one-third of those having hip replacements. In 1991, University of Cincinnati researchers tried giving aspirin instead. Starting the night before their surgery and continuing twice a day afterward for two weeks, 177 new-hip recipients took 650 mg of aspirin (two standard tablets). None developed heterotopic ossification. The researchers concluded, "Aspirin is a safe and inexpensive agent for prevention of [this complication]."

ASPIRIN MIGHT EVEN HELP TREAT LEPROSY

Leprosy was a scourge during biblical times. Those with the disfiguring disease were banished to prisonlike leper colonies, and even today the term *leper* means outcast. Leprosy is a chronic bacterial infection that causes skin discoloration and, in severe cases, blindness and crippling of the hands. Also called Hansen's disease, leprosy is rare in the United

States—about 5,000 Americans have it—but worldwide an estimated 15 million people are infected.

Leprosy is difficult to treat, although new drugs have shown promise and several vaccines are being developed. Recently, a British researcher suggested that prostaglandins might play a role in the development of the disease, and that as a prostaglandin-inhibitor, aspirin might help treat it. He suggested a clinical trial: "There is little to lose by trying—and a great deal to gain."

CHAPTER SEVEN

. . . AND DON'T FORGET ASPIRIN FOR PAIN, FEVER, AND INFLAMMATION

~~~~~

Aspirin's preventive uses have generated headlines, but they account for only a small fraction of its uses. Most people still take aspirin to treat fever, headache, arthritis, and the pain of common household, occupational, and athletic injuries. The commercials call aspirin "the pain reliever doctors recommend most," and with a few important exceptions discussed in this chapter and in Chapter 9, that statement remains as true today as ever.

ASPIRIN VERSUS FEVER

Fever is an oral temperature of 100°F (37.8°C) or higher, a rectal temperature of 101°F (38.3°C), or an underarm (axillary) temperature of 98.6°F (37.0°C).

Fever usually means that the body is fighting an infection. Body temperature, however, has a daily cycle—lowest around 3:00 A.M., highest in the late afternoon—and other factors can raise body temperature close to the fever point: immunizations, strenuous exercise, and some medications.

Most people consider fever "bad," something to get rid of as quickly as possible. In fact, fever is of considerable value in fighting infection. Most disease-causing microorganisms have difficulty reproducing at temperatures much above normal body temperature, so fever evolved as one of the ways the immune system fights them. When cells become infected, they release special chemicals (endogenous pyrogens) that tell the brain to increase body temperature. The immune system's white blood cells also signal the brain to turn up the body's thermostat, located in the part of the brain called the "hypothalamus."

Scientists are not completely sure how the body raises its temperature, but the leading theory is that endogenous pyrogens increase the level of one family of prostaglandins in the blood, prostaglandin E, which in turn raises the body's thermostat. The strongest evidence in favor of this theory is that drugs that inhibit prostaglandin synthesis, including aspirin, also reduce fever (antipyretics).

Because fever is one of the immune system's weapons against infection, some physicians suggest *not* treating it unless it reaches 102° in children or 101° in adults, or unless it causes significant discomfort and/or insomnia. There is currently no convincing evidence that reducing fever interferes with the immune system or lengthens the duration of infectious diseases. Whether or not you treat your fevers, drink plenty of nonalcoholic liquids to replace fluids lost through the increase in perspiration caused by elevated temperature.

To treat fevers with aspirin, take two standard tablets (650 mg) every four hours. Aspirin begins to reduce fever within 30 to 60 minutes and attains its maximum temperature-reducing effect within two to three hours. For faster action, crush the tablets and dissolve them in water.

Aspirin typically reduces fever 2° to 3°F, so it usually brings low-grade fevers down to normal but may not normalize unusually high fevers.

At a dose of 650 mg every four hours, aspirin may cause several side effects: stomach distress, gastrointestinal bleeding, increased bruising and clotting time, ringing in the ears (tinnitus), allergic reactions, and/or gout attacks. When in doubt about the advisability of taking aspirin, consult a physician.

Aspirin side effects, discussed in Chapter 8, are a major reason why so many Americans treat fever with acetaminophen or ibuprofen, whose fever-fighting action is approximately equivalent to aspirin's. (See Chapter 9 for a comparison of these three drugs.)

Never give aspirin to a child under 18 for a fever associated with colds, flu, or chickenpox. It may cause Reye's syndrome, a rare but potentially fatal condition affecting the brain and liver. Of course, it's often difficult to tell if a feverish child has a cold or flu. As a result, many physicians advise against treating childhood fevers with aspirin, period. For more on aspirin and children, see Chapter 10.

Some fevers require professional care. Call a physician for:

- Any fever in a pregnant woman
- Any fever in anyone with heart disease, chronic respiratory disease, or any serious chronic medical condition
- Any fever that lasts longer than five days (three days in children)
- Any fever that does not respond to home treatment within thirty-six hours
- Any fever that initially responds to treatment, then recurs
- If signs of dehydration develop—extreme thirst, light-headedness, infrequent or dark urine, dry mouth, and decreased skin elasticity (Risk of dehydration is highest in children and the elderly.)

Consult a physician *immediately* if fever is accompanied by a rash, severe headache, stiff neck, marked irritability or confusion, cough with brown/green sputum, severe back or abdominal pain, or painful urination. Fever and any of these signs may indicate a potentially serious illness—pneumonia or meningitis, among others.

ASPIRIN VERSUS PAIN

Nobel Prize–winning physician Albert Schweitzer called pain "a more terrible Lord over humanity than even Death himself." Pain is the leading reason why people consult physicians. And no wonder. According to a 1985 Lou Harris survey, here's the painful truth about what British poet Sir William Watson (1858–1935) called "the monster with a thousand teeth":

Type of Pain	Americans reporting it in 1984 (%)
Headache	73
Back pain	56
Muscle aches and pains	53
Joint pain	51
Stomach pain	46
Menstrual cramps	40
Dental pain	27

Of those reporting back, joint, and muscle pain, more than 10 percent were in pain for at least a hundred days of the survey year. The only type of pain that does not lend itself to treatment with aspirin is stomach pain, which the drug might aggravate.

Most people understand pain to be bioelectrical. Damaged cells stimulate pain-sensing nerves, which relay an electrical message to the brain that something hurts.

Pain is also biochemical. Damaged cells release several chemicals crucial to pain perception. They trigger inflammation and "sensitize" the pain-sensing nerves. To appreciate sensitization, consider how it feels to pull on a pair of pants at the beach. Some sand in the pants causes little discomfort. But if your legs are sunburned, injured skin cells release the sensitizing chemicals, and pulling on sandy pants may feel like torture. One of the most potent pain-sensitizing families of chemicals are the prostaglandins. Aspirin's antiprostaglandin action is the reason it relieves pain. (Ibuprofen is also a prostaglandin inhibitor.)

A study published in the journal *Science* in late 1992 suggests that aspirin also relieves pain by blocking the transmission of pain messages among certain spinal nerves—at least in rats. Researchers at the University of California at San Diego injected aspirin into the spinal cords of rats. By measuring substances produced when these animals are in pain, the researchers deduced that the injections produced significantly more pain relief than would have resulted from the same dose of aspirin taken by mouth. This animal study is preliminary—and its applicability to humans remains to be investigated—but it raises the exciting possibility that one day inexpensive, nonaddictive aspirin might be used as a pain-relieving substitute for today's strongest, more costly analgesics, the addictive narcotics. This research also shows that scientists still have a great deal to learn about aspirin's role in pain relief.

To treat pain with aspirin, take two standard tablets (650 mg) every four hours. Aspirin begins to relieve pain within 30 to 60 minutes, and attains its maximum effect within two to three hours. For faster action, crush the tablets in water.

Aspirin's major side effects are mentioned in the "Fever"

section of this chapter, and discussed more fully in Chapter 8. When in doubt about the advisability of taking aspirin, consult a physician.

Acetaminophen and ibuprofen also relieve pain. Their analgesic action is similar to aspirin's, but for reasons that remain unclear, several studies show that ibuprofen is superior for treating menstrual cramps.

Injured children who do not have fevers may be treated with aspirin. For dosage recommendations, see Chapter 10.

Consult a physician if:

- Aspirin (or any analgesic) does not relieve pain substantially within two weeks
- Pain becomes more severe despite home treatment
- Other symptoms develop in addition to pain: fever, fainting, confusion, vision disturbances, skin discoloration, bone or joint deformities, or loss of mobility or range of motion.

ASPIRIN VERSUS INFLAMMATION

Pain does not necessarily cause inflammation, but significant inflammation almost always causes pain. Inflammation also produces redness, swelling, warmth, and opening of the small blood vessels (capillary dilation), which brings into the area extra blood carrying white blood cells and immune proteins to fight whatever is causing the inflammation: an injury, irritant, infection, allergy, or anything that stimulates an immune response, sometimes even the body's own tissues in autoimmune diseases such as rheumatoid arthritis.

Scientists are not entirely certain how aspirin relieves inflammation, but the immune system releases type-E prostaglandins at cellular injury sites. Presumably, prostaglandin inhibition accounts for at least part of aspirin's (and ibuprofen's) antiinflammatory action.

The inflammatory condition most frequently treated with aspirin is joint inflammation, or arthritis, which affects some 37 million Americans. Most people associate it with aging. The prevalence of arthritis does increase with age, but it strikes people of all ages. "Arthritis" is not a single disease but rather a symptom of literally dozens of illnesses, everything from mumps and tuberculosis to syphilis and Lyme disease. The two most common forms are osteoarthritis and rheumatoid arthritis.

Osteoarthritis, also known as degenerative joint disease, is by far the leading cause of joint inflammation. More than half of adults over age thirty suffer from it to some extent. Osteoarthritis develops when the tough, flexible, shock-absorbing cartilage in the joints, which keeps the bones from grinding against one another, breaks down or becomes inflamed. Any joint can develop osteoarthritis, with overuse and previous injury often preceding its development. The main symptoms are pain, stiffness, and often, though not always, inflammation. Usually the pain is an aching associated with movement of the affected joint(s). It typically subsides when the joint is rested. Some osteoarthritis sufferers experience morning stiffness, which usually subsides with movement during the day.

Rheumatoid arthritis is the most crippling form of joint disease, affecting some 6 million Americans. Unlike osteoarthritis, which generally develops among older adults, rheumatoid arthritis can strike at any age, even during infancy, although it's most likely to occur between 30 and 40. Its cause remains unclear, but most researchers consider it an autoimmune condition—the body's own immune system attacks the joints and causes the pain, inflammation, and deformities. The major symptoms are pain, stiffness, redness, and swelling. The joints most commonly affected are in the hands and feet, which may become severely deformed. The pain is often severe, and unlike osteoarthritis, it does not subside with rest.

Some people self-medicate their osteoarthritis or rheumatoid arthritis with aspirin (or over-the-counter ibuprofen). Others prefer one of the many prescription nonsteroidal antiinflammatory drugs: naproxen (Naprosyn, Anaprox), flurbiprofen (Ansaid), sulindac (Clinoril), ibuprofen (Motrin), or indomethacin (Indocin, Indameth), among others. Compared with aspirin, NSAIDs cost a great deal more, but studies show that they do not provide substantially better relief of pain and inflammation. "Despite the development of newer anti-inflammatory agents," the latest edition of a leading pharmacology text says, "aspirin is still regarded as the standard against which other drugs should be compared." And in a recent article in the journal *Rheumatic Disease Clinics,* researchers at the Medical College of Wisconsin at Milwaukee reached the same conclusion, arguing that physicians and arthritis sufferers "hold aspirin in low esteem" because unlike the newer prescription NSAIDs, it's an over-the-counter drug, which implies that it's less effective. Not so. "In our experience, aspirin remains the most consistently effective NSAID available for the treatment of rheumatoid arthritis."

Aspirin provides antiinflammatory benefits only at relatively high doses. As little as 30 mg a day help prevent stroke; the Physicians' Health Study showed that 325 mg every other day help prevent heart attack; most headaches clear up with 650 mg (two tablets). But for the pain and inflammation of adult rheumatoid arthritis, the recommended dose is 5,000 to 8,000 mg a day (up to 24 standard tablets a day).

At such high doses, side effects are almost inevitable, particularly gastrointestinal distress and bleeding. For more on aspirin side effects, see Chapter 8. Prescription NSAIDs have similar side effects, but people react to drugs differently. For physicians, one of the challenges of managing arthritis is to find an effective antiinflammatory whose side effects the person can tolerate. For some, aspirin works best. Other experience greater relief and fewer side effects from ibuprofen (in either over-the-counter or prescription strength), or from a prescription NSAID.

Arthritis requires ongoing professional care. It's also a good idea to contact the Arthritis Foundation (1314 Spring Street, N.W., Atlanta, GA 30309; [404] 872-7100), which publishes helpful information, and sponsors self-help groups around the country. For the chapter nearest you, contact the national office or consult your phone book. Studies show that arthritis sufferers who learn about the condition, and adapt to it, lead more normal lives and require less pain medication than those who remain uninformed or give in to despair.

Contact a physician if:

- Joint pain becomes significantly worse despite home treatment, or if
- You develop a single warm, swollen, painful joint, which suggests an infection (septic arthritis)

TOPICAL ASPIRIN VERSUS CALLUSES AND INSECT STINGS

"Topical" means applied to the skin surface. For the vast majority of its uses, aspirin must be absorbed into the bloodstream, but not for treatment of calluses and insect stings.

Calluses are raised, usually painless bumps of dead skin that develop on the hands, toes, bottoms of the feet, or anywhere the skin is subjected to friction over time. They develop to protect the sensitive underlayer of skin (dermis), and in general should not be disturbed. But sometimes calluses become unsightly, or grow uncomfortably large.

Some doctors say that calluses can be reduced in size by applying a paste of five crushed aspirin tablets and one tablespoon of lemon juice mixed with one tablespoon of water.

Both aspirin and lemon juice are acidic, and the paste made from these two mild acids helps soften callused skin. Apply the paste generously, then cover the callus with a bandage or plastic bag for 15 to 30 minutes. After the skin has softened, use a pumice stone or metal file to remove the outer layer of callus tissue. Repeat two to three times a week until the callus has been reduced to the desired size.

A few physicians, among them Australian Richard J. Von Witt, also endorse the folk remedy of rubbing an aspirin tablet into insect stings for relief of pain and inflammation. Here's the recommendation he published in 1980 in *The Lancet:*

> The [inflammation, pain], itching, and irritation caused by insect stings can be considerably reduced by the use of a topically applied solution of aspirin. Moisten the area of the sting, then apply a coating of aspirin by rubbing a [tablet] onto the area. When the initial relief has passed, the aspirin can be moistened again and the effect will persist. It seems likely that topical aspirin is sufficient to dampen the inflammatory reaction and provide local analgesia. I do not suggest this simple treatment for people with severe allergies [to aspirin, but it] usually helps calm others and does not have the side effects of antihistamines.

A FDA advisory panel on pain relief considered aspirin for insect bites and stings but concluded that the evidence was insufficient to recommend it as a topical analgesic. If you get bitten or stung, assuming you're not allergic, there's no harm in rubbing on some powdered aspirin. It just might help.

NOT RECOMMENDED: TOPICAL ASPIRIN
FOR SORE THROAT OR TOOTHACHE

While aspirin helps insect stings, its topical benefits do not, apparently, extend to gargling aspirin and water for a sore throat, or rubbing tablets on teeth that ache. Unlike stings, sore throat and toothache are not really surface phenomena. The pain usually results from infection of underlying tissue. Aspirin might relieve sore throat and toothache pain, but only if the drug gets into the bloodstream—so swallow it.

On the other hand, for the sore throat of the common cold, few physicians recommend aspirin. They suggest drinking hot liquids and/or sucking on hard candies or anesthetic throat lozenges. For sore throat with fever, but no other cold symptoms, consult a physician. It might be strep throat, which might require antibiotics.

For any toothache or tooth sensitivity, consult a dentist. You might have a cavity, a cracked or chipped tooth, or a problem with a filling. Rubbing an aspirin against an aching tooth might actually cause harm. The rubbing might injure gum tissue.

CHAPTER EIGHT

ASPIRIN SIDE EFFECTS AND INTERACTIONS

Aspirin's hundred-year history as an over-the-counter family favorite has lulled many people into thinking it's harmless. It isn't. Aspirin's amazing medical benefits come at the price of sometimes significant—and for some people, hazardous—side effects. Most people can take low preventive doses and moderate therapeutic doses safely, but everyone should still understand this drug's side effects and interactions, and recognize the signs that mean it's time to take less or discontinue it.

OVERDOSE

More than 10,000 Americans overdose on aspirin each year. Most recover simply by discontinuing the drug, but hundreds develop aspirin intoxication, low-level poisoning that often requires medical treatment, and dozens suffer serious aspirin poisoning, a potentially fatal medical emergency. Despite childproof containers, aspirin remains one of the leading causes of childhood poisoning deaths.

Aspirin has caused death in adults at doses of 10 to 30 grams (30 to 90 standard tablets). The lethal dose in children is 150 mg/kg, or about 70 mg/lb. For a 65-pound child, the lethal dose would be approximately 4.5 g (14 standard tablets). Aspirin intoxication and poisoning may develop at lower doses. In fact, in both children and adults who take it regularly over time for such conditions as rheumatoid arthritis, therapeutic doses can cause real problems.

The symptoms of aspirin intoxication (salicylism) include:

- Dizziness
- Headache
- Ringing in the ears (tinnitus)
- Difficulty hearing
- Severe abdominal pain
- Nausea
- Vomiting
- Diarrhea
- Confusion
- Lethargy
- Anxiety

Aspirin poisoning causes these same symptoms plus:

- Rapid breathing (hyperventilation)
- Rapid heartbeat (tachycardia)
- Fever (especially in children)
- Sweating
- Thirst
- Dimness of vision
- Hallucinations

- Delerium
- Convulsions
- Coma

If you suspect aspirin intoxication or poisoning, call 911 immediately and follow the operator's instructions. To eliminate as much aspirin as possible, the 911 operator might advise you to induce vomiting with syrup of ipecac followed by water. Administer the dose the operator recommends. Every home medicine chest should contain syrup of ipecac. If yours does not, add it to your shopping list *now*. The 911 operator might also advise you to give activated charcoal for aspirin overdose in young children. First-aid kits often contain this item, or ask for it at your pharmacy.

Of course, overdose prevention is preferable to emergency first aid. Make sure elderly loved ones—especially those with arthritis who take aspirin regularly—understand its possible toxicity. People with arthritis of the hands often have difficulty opening childproof containers. They may store aspirin and other medicines in more easily opened boxes and jars. There's nothing wrong with this—unless young children visit. If you have young children, be aware that the homes of friends and relatives, particularly their medicine cabinets and under-sink areas, may not be childproof.

Childproof containers have greatly reduced accidental childhood poisonings, but they still occur, and aspirin still ranks high among the drugs that poison children. Why? Because childproof containers have an unpublicized but possibly fatal flaw. Some children can open them with their teeth. The smaller the diameter of the container cap, the easier it is for children to bite it off. If you have young children, or if they visit you, buy aspirin and other medicines packaged in containers with the largest caps you can find. And always keep drug containers out of the reach of children.

Even at moderate doses, aspirin may contribute to salicylism if other drugs and/or food additives containing salicylates are consumed at the same time. Drugs containing salicylates include: Pepto-Bismol (bismuth subsalicylate); Magan, Magsal, and Trilisate (magnesium salicylate); Pabalate-SF (potassium salicylate); Disalcid, Mono-Gesic, and Salflex (salsalate); and the many brand-name pain relievers that contain aspirin: Alka-Seltzer, Anacin, Excedrin, and Vanquish, among others. If the label or your pharmacist says the drug contains ASA, acetylsalicylic acid, salsalate, or anything with salicylates, it's a form of aspirin and may contribute to an overdose.

STOMACH UPSET

Anyone who has ever seen a Tylenol or Bufferin commercial knows that aspirin can upset the stomach. About 5 percent of those who take therapeutic doses of aspirin to treat everyday aches and pains experience heartburn, abdominal distress, nausea, or vomiting. An estimated one-third to two-thirds of aspirin consumers notice mild to moderate abdominal discomfort. The low doses of aspirin used to prevent heart attack and stroke cause fewer stomach problems, but among participants in the studies discussed in Chapters 1 and 2, complaints of abdominal distress were by no means rare.

There are several ways to prevent aspirin-related stomach distress:

• Take it after eating. Aspirin is less likely to cause irritation when it's not the only thing in the stomach.
• Crush it and mix with water or another nonalcoholic liquid, for example fruit juice. In solution, aspirin passes into the intestine faster and has less time to irritate the stomach.
• Take an enteric-coated brand (Ecotrin, Halfprin). Several studies show that the coating protects the stomach lining. The main disadvantages are cost and delayed action.

• Take it with an antacid. Ever since Bristol-Meyers began marketing its aspirin-antacid combination, Bufferin, in 1949, its advertising has claimed that it "helps prevent the stomach upset often caused by aspirin." But in 1971, a panel of the National Academy of Sciences and National Research Council reviewed dozens of studies on the subject and found "little difference in the incidence or intensity of gastrointestinal side effects after ingestion of Bufferin or plain aspirin." Neither Bufferin nor generic buffered aspirin contain much antacid. On the other hand, they might have enough to make a difference to you. If so, generic buffered aspirin is considerably cheaper than Bufferin.

For stronger buffering action, try taking aspirin with one of the many over-the-counter antacids (Di-Gel, Gelusil, Maalox, Remegel, Riopan, Rolaids, and Tums, among others). Yet, according to one recent study, even these products do not provide reliable relief. If you have high blood pressure, consult your physician or pharmacist before using antacids.

For maximum protection, take an antacid with enteric-coated aspirin after meals. If you still suffer stomach distress, try acetaminophen, or consult a physician.

The stomach may not be the only part of the upper GI tract irritated by aspirin. Above it sits the esophagus, which can become painfully inflamed (esophagitis). In a recent study of 186 esophagitis patients at the University of Alabama, prior aspirin use turned out to be the only significant risk factor.

BLEEDING

Aspirin's anticlotting action is the reason it helps prevent heart attack, stroke, and several other conditions discussed in this book. But increased clotting time has a definite downside. In normal individuals, the standard two-tablet (650 mg) therapeutic dose of aspirin approximately doubles the time it takes blood to clot. The effect of a single therapeutic dose may last up to several days. In the case of shaving nicks, this is a minor annoyance—and a small price to pay for aspirin's remarkable preventive value. For some people, however, the cost of slower clotting may outweigh the benefits. Those with the following concerns should consult a physician about the advisability of using aspirin:

Surgery. Most physicians advise against taking aspirin for a week before surgery to reduce the risk of postoperative bleeding complications.

Dental extractions. Most dentists make the same recommendation for the same reason.

Clotting disorders. Hemophilia, von Willebrand's disease, or any other clotting disorder may preclude use of aspirin. If you have one ask your physician or pharmacist about the advisability of taking aspirin.

Anticoagulants. If you take any anticoagulant medications, consult your physician or pharmacist before taking aspirin.

Hemorrhagic conditions. From chronic nosebleeds to cerebral hemorrhage, if you have any bleeding disorder, consult your physician or pharmacist before taking aspirin.

A tendency to bruise easily. Bruising is caused by bleeding under the skin. If you bruise easily, consult your physician or pharmacist about the advisability of taking aspirin.

Red spots in the whites of your eyes. These are medically known as subconjunctival hematomas, and they indicate minor bleeding in the eye. They are usually harmless but can be frightening and cause cosmetic problems. If you experience this problem frequently, ask your physician about the advisability of taking aspirin.

Vitamin K deficiency. This vitamin is necessary for normal clotting. If you're deficient, consult your physician or pharmacist before taking aspirin.

Few people are aware that some foods have an anticlotting effect that might add to aspirin's. Chief among them are garlic and coldwater fish high in omega-3 fatty acids: salmon, tuna, mackerel, sardines, herring, bluefish, and trout. Diets high in garlic and omega-3 fatty acids have been associated with a decreased risk of heart attack, but those who take aspirin regularly should be aware of a possible synergistic effect of regular aspirin use and a diet containing these foods.

GASTROINTESTINAL BLEEDING

In the normal course of digestion, everyone experiences a tiny amount of gastrointestinal (GI) bleeding. This blood loss is painless and typically amounts to about 0.6 ml per day—about one-tenth of a teaspoon. Aspirin damages the stomach lining (gastric mucosa), and any use increases GI bleeding. Aspirin-induced GI bleeding is also painless, but those with gastroinestinal diseases—such as ulcers, colitis, or Crohn's disease—should consult their physicians about the advisability of taking the drug.

For those with normal GI tracts, low-dose aspirin use rarely causes significant GI bleeding. Higher-dose occasional therapeutic use causes more bleeding, but again, it's usually not a problem.

Aspirin-related GI bleeding becomes a problem only for those who use therapeutic doses regularly (at least four days a week) for treatment of chronic headaches, sprains, tendinitis, muscle injuries, and arthritis. Rheumatoid arthritis sufferers, who may consume large amounts of aspirin regularly, are at highest risk. In one study, a daily lose of 4 to 5 g of aspirin a day (12 to 16 standard tablets) multiplied GI bleeding tenfold, up to about one teaspoon.

Regular consumption of alcohol also increases aspirin-related GI bleeding.

One concern with aspirin-related GI bleeding is the possibility of iron-deficiency anemia. Physicians caring for rheumatoid arthritis sufferers may perform periodic blood tests to check blood iron levels.

Another more serious concern is the risk of developing or aggravating ulcers. Risk factors for aspirin-induced ulcers include: large doses, age over 60, a history of ulcers or other GI problems, and regular use of alcohol, cigarettes, or corticosteroid drugs. If you take therapeutic doses of aspirin regularly and have any of these risk factors, discuss your ulcer risk with your physician.

Occasionally, those who take large doses of aspirin regularly suffer massive GI bleeding. They either vomit blood (hematemesis) or show large amounts in their stool (melena). These problems are medical emergencies. An estimated one-third of those hospitalized with these conditions are regular aspirin users. Many are alcoholics.

Until recently, physicians could not prevent aspirin-related GI bleeding, but now three approaches show promise—red (cayenne) pepper, ranitidine (Zantac), and misoprostol (Cytotec). Red pepper's fiery taste comes from the chemical capsaicin. The myth is that spicy foods contribute to ulcers, but recent research has shown that capsaicin causes no harm—and might even be protective. In a 1989 animal study, capsaicin prevented aspirin-related GI bleeding and ulcer formation. This effect has not been demonstrated in humans, but if you'd like to try capsaicin and don't have any GI problems, many supplement and health food stores sell red pepper capsules.

A 1988 study showed that 150 mg of ranitidine prevented GI bleeding and ulcer formation in those who took 15 aspirins (five 900 mg doses) over a two-day period. A 1991 German study confirmed these results. If you're interested in ranitidine, discuss it with your physician.

Several studies also show that misoprostol substantially reduces aspirin-related GI bleeding and ulcer formation. If you're interested in this medication, consult your physician.

HEARING

Large doses of aspirin may cause ringing in the ears (tinnitus) and hearing impairment. These side effects are symptoms of aspirin overdose, but in some people they may develop even at moderate therapeutic doses. Aspirin affects hearing by altering the way the hair cells in the inner ear transmit auditory signals. In most cases, ringing and hearing loss clear up within two to three days after discontinuing aspirin. But a 1989 animal study at the University of North Carolina suggests that the combination of large doses of aspirin and loud noise might add up to permanent hearing impairment. If you have tinnitus or any hearing problem, ask your physician about the advisability of taking aspirin.

SENSITIVITY: ASTHMA AND HIVES

In about three people per thousand, aspirin precipitates the wheezing and bronchial spasms of asthma or the red welt eruptions of hives. Among those with asthma or chronic hives, the risk of allergic reaction is much higher—around 20 percent. Occasionally, within minutes after taking aspirin, someone with aspirin-sensitive asthma or hives develops the rapidly life-threatening reaction known as anaphylaxis, a medical emergency involving rapid onset of difficult breathing. Anyone who develops breathing difficulties shortly after taking aspirin should be rushed to an emergency room.

The cause of aspirin sensitivity remains unclear, but it has been extensively documented since 1902. Most of those sensitive to aspirin are also sensitive to several other nonsteroidal antiinflammatory drugs, among them ibuprofen, indomethacin, naproxen, and sulindac. A few are also sensitive to acetaminophen. Fortunately, many of those sensitive to aspirin can be desensitized by exposure to gradually increased doses.

Those with asthma or chronic hives should discuss the possibility of aspirin sensitivity with their physicians, and request a "nasal challenge" test to see if they are sensitive. This test involves inhaling a small amount of powdered aspirin to see if it provokes a reaction. (Nasal challenge reactions tend to be mild.) Those who are aspirin sensitive should not take aspirin or other salicylates until they have been desensitized because of the risk of anaphylaxis, which can be rapidly fatal.

GOUT

Anyone with a history of gout should consult a physician about the advisability of taking aspirin. The drug may precipitate gout attacks.

Gout is a form of arthritis. It causes inflammation and often intense pain in one or more joints, most commonly the big toe. Gout is caused by the buildup of uric acid, a metabolic waste product that is a component of urine. Normally, the kidneys filter uric acid out of the blood, but in people with gout, some gets deposited as crystals in the joints. A gout attack occurs when these crystals irritate the joint lining. Aspirin may increase blood levels of uric acid, and interfere with the effectiveness of the drugs used to treat gout (probenecid and sulfinpyrazone).

MACULAR DEGENERATION

Macular degeneration is a leading cause of vision impairment and blindness in the elderly. The macula is the part of the eye's nerve-rich retina that distinguishes fine detail at the center of the field of vision. With age, the blood vessels that supply the macula may deteriorate to the point where central vision becomes blurry or worse. Peripheral vision is not affected.

Some physicians have expressed concern that aspirin's antiplatelet action might contribute to macular bleeding and aggravate any degeneration. This possibility raises a potentially serious issue because those at greatest risk for macular degeneration, older adults, are the same people most likely to benefit from aspirin's ability to prevent heart attack and ischemic stroke.

As this book goes to press, surprisingly few studies have investigated this question. The largest and best to date, an evaluation of 732 people with macular degeneration, showed no differences in eye bleeding between those who took aspirin regularly and those who did not. Writing in the *Journal of the American Medical Association,* Michael Klein, of the Oregon Health Sciences University, commented: "Current data do not support the hypothesis of an increased incidence of hemorrhage associated with the use of aspirin in patients with age-related macular degeneration."

On the other hand, if you have macular degeneration, consult your physician about the advisability of taking aspirin regularly.

VITAMIN AND MINERAL INTERACTIONS

Don't take aspirin and vitamin C at the same time. In combination, they increase the likelihood of stomach upset.

Aspirin may also interfere with the absorption of vitamin C, folic acid, and iron. If you take aspirin regularly, supplementation with these nutrients might be advisable. If stomach upset results, take aspirin and vitaminc C at separate times.

DRUG INTERACTIONS

In addition to the gout drugs mentioned above, aspirin also interacts with many others.

Alcohol. As mentioned earlier, alcohol increases aspirin-induced stomach upset. One recent study shows that compared with the blood-alcohol level achieved from drinking alone, the combination of therapeutic doses of aspirin and alcohol results in blood-alcohol levels that are significantly higer—with a risk of significantly increased intoxication. Two other similar studies showed no such increase. This question remains open, but it would be prudent to exercise caution when combining aspirin and alcohol.

Antacids. These drugs may do more than decrease aspirin-induced stomach upset. They may reduce its effectiveness as well by increasing its rate of excretion.

Beta-blockers, ACE inhibitors, and loop diuretics. Aspirin may decrease the effectiveness of these blood pressure medications. If you take one, consult your physician or pharmacist about the advisability of taking aspirin at the same time.

Corticosteroids. These antiinflammatory drugs increase the rate of aspirin excretion and may decrease its pain-relieving action. Corticosteroids include the dozens of brands of: cortisone, hydrocortisone, prednisone, prednisolone, triamcinolone, methylprednisolone, paramethasone, dexamethasone, and betamethasone. If you take a corticosteroid, consult your physician or pharmacist about the advisability of taking aspirin at the same time.

Diuretics. Among the many different types of diuretics, the carbonic anhydrase inhibitors—Daranide, Diamox, AK-Zol, Neptazane, and Acetazolamide—may increase the risk of aspirin intoxication. If you take this type of diuretic, consult your physician or pharmacist about the advisability of taking aspirin at the same time.

Insulin and sulfonylureas. These drugs are used to control blood glucose levels in diabetics. Aspirin in doses greater than 2 g per day (about six standard tablets) reduces blood glucose and may increase the effects of insulin and many sulfonylurea medications. If you have diabetes, consult your physician or pharmacist about the advisability of taking aspirin in combination with any diabetes medication.

Methotrexate. This drug is used to treat rheumatoid arthritis (Rheumatrex), psoriasis (Folex, Abitrexate), and several cancers (Mexate). Simultaneous use of aspirin may increase methotrexate blood levels. If you take this drug, consult your physician or pharmacist about the advisability of taking aspirin at the same time.

Nitroglycerin. Nitroglycerin is used to control angina. A few studies suggest that simultaneous use of aspirin may cause a significant drop in blood pressure and possibly fainting. If you take nitroglycerin, consult your physician or pharmacist about the advisability of taking aspirin at the same time.

Nonsteroidal antiinflammatory drugs (NSAIDs).
These drugs have aspirinlike analgesic and antiinflammatory effects. Combined with aspirin, risk of stomach upset increases.

Valproic acid.
Simultaneous use of aspirin increases blood levels of this antiseizure drug, increasing its effect. Brands include: Depakene, Deproic, Depa, Depakote, and Myproic Acid. If you take valproic acid, consult your physician or pharmacist about the advisability of taking aspirin at the same time.

Aspirin may interact with other drugs as well. If you take any medication regularly, consult your physician or pharmacist about the advisability of taking aspirin at the same time.

DIAGNOSTIC TEST INTERACTIONS

The most important of these is the occult blood test for colorectal cancer (see Chapter 4). Before early-stage colorectal tumors cause symptoms, they release a tiny amount of blood, which is invisible (occult) to the eye but detectable using a chemical test. The American Cancer Society recommends an occult blood test annually for everyone over age 50. Because aspirin causes gastrointestinal bleeding, aspirin use shortly before an occult blood test may produce an erroneous positive result (false positive). Physicians typically recommend refraining from aspirin use for several days—sometimes up to a week—before occult blood testing.

Aspirin may affect other diagnostic tests as well. If you take aspirin frequently, mention it to your physician before any medical test.

CHAPTER NINE

ASPIRIN VERSUS THE COMPETITION

Tylenol, Bufferin, Anacin, Excedrin, Advil, Motrin. It's difficult to turn on a TV or open a newspaper or magazine without seeing advertisements for these and many other aspirin competitors. Low-dose aspirin is the *only one* shown to prevent heart attack, stroke, and the other conditions discussed in Chapters 1 through 6. In addition, the experts agree that in therapeutic doses, no aspirin competitor is substantially better for relief of fever, pain, and inflammation. But several distinctions are worth mentioning:

- Aspirin and ibuprofen (Advil, Motrin, etc.) relieve inflammation; acetaminophen (Tylenol, etc.) does not.
- Acetaminophen causes less stomach upset than aspirin and ibuprofen.
- Ibuprofen provides the best relief of menstrual cramps and dental pain.

- Aspirin should not be given to children for treatment of fever. Acetaminophen is the drug of choice (see Chapter 10).
- The latest research suggests that aspirin-caffeine combinations may relieve pain somewhat more effectively than plain aspirin.

THE OTHER ASPIRINS

Aspirin by any other name is still aspirin. It just costs more. The most heavily advertised brands include: Alka-Seltzer (all forms), Anacin, Arthritis Pain Formula, Bayer, Bufferin (all forms), Ecotrin, Emprin, and Excedrin. In addition, there are about a dozen other brands: A.S.A., Ascriptin, Asperbuf, Aspercin, Aspergum, Aspermin, Aspirtab, Buff-A, Buffaprin, Buffasal, Cosprin, Measurin, Momentum, and St. Joseph among others. Some are simply aspirin; others are chewable, enteric-coated, or time-released. Some are buffered with antacids and others contain what the commercials never tire of calling "a combination of ingredients."

Simply aspirin. These products include Aspercin, Aspermin, Aspertab, Bayer aspirin, Cosprin, Emprin, and Norwich aspirin. All aspirin must be manufactured to the same FDA standards, so despite their advertising claims, no brand is either "purer" or "more trustworthy" than generic aspirin. Doan's Pills, promoted for back pain, contain magnesium salicylate, which, for all practical purposes, is aspirin.

Chewable, enteric-coated, time-released. Back in the 1950s, chewable Aspergum was what led Lawrence Craven to speculate on aspirin's ability to prevent heart attack. But it's difficult to come up with a good reason to use it today. Those who have difficulty swallowing aspirin tablets can simply crush them and mix them with water or juice.

Some people think Aspergum helps relieve the pain of tooth-aches, canker sores, and sore throats. It does—but only after it passes through the stomach and is absorbed into the blood-stream. Except in the case of insect stings, aspirin is not a surface-acting (topical) pain reliever.

Enteric-coated aspirin (Ecotrin, Halfprin, etc.) helps pre-vent stomach upset because the coating doesn't dissolve until the pill has left the stomach. It's a reasonable alternative for those with unusually aspirin-sensitive stomachs or people with arthritis who take large doses regularly. For the occasional aspirin user, minor stomach distress can usually be prevented by taking generic aspirin after meals and/or by crushing and mixing with water or juice so that it passes out of the stom-ach more quickly than it does in solid pill form.

Enteric-coatings are good but not perfect. Occasionally they dissolve prematurely in the stomach, which sabotages the reason for using it. Occasionally they don't dissolve at all when passing through the digestive tract. The pill comes out whole, which means no fever, pain, or inflammation relief. Finally, coated aspirin also takes longer to begin working—about 60 minutes as opposed to approximately 15 minutes for uncoated aspirin.

Time-released aspirin can be taken every eight to 12 hours instead of every four. This might be a boon at bedtime for all-night pain relief, but the added convenience has a few costs. Time-released aspirin is more expensive than generic aspirin, and the delayed release depends on coatings similar to those on enteric-coated aspirin. The ads tout the steady flow of aspirin into the bloodstream, but release may be er-ratic, resulting in peaks and valleys of aspirin blood levels. Whenever possible, experts recommend taking two regular tablets every four hours.

Buffered. Buffers are antacids that supposedly help pre-vent aspirin-induced stomach distress. As discussed in Chap-ter 8, however, the research shows that Bufferin—and other buffered brands—are not significantly gentler to the stomach than plain aspirin. They don't contain enough antacid to have much soothing action. To minimize stomach upset, take aspirin on a full stomach, or crush and mix with water or juice. Or take an enteric-coated brand or an over-the-counter antacid along with your aspirin.

For years, Bufferin advertising also made the claim it "works twice as fast as plain aspirin." The same 1971 National Academy of Sciences–National Research Council panel that shot down Bufferin's claim of gentleness also took the product to task for its claim of greater speed. Some buffered aspirins are, in fact, absorbed into the bloodstream faster than plain aspirin, but not *twice* as fast, and according to the panel, "there is no evidence to indicate that [increased speed of absorption] significantly increases speed of onset of action." In 1986, the American Pharmaceutical Association came to the same conclusion in its authoritative *Handbook of Nonprescription Drugs:* "There is no evidence from controlled clinical studies that buffered aspirin provides more rapid onset or a greater degree of pain relief than nonbuffered aspirin."

The one possible exception is Alka-Seltzer, the popular effervescent buffered aspirin, which might provide noticeably more rapid action because in addition to being buffered it's also dissolved in water, which increases speed of absorption. The problem with Alka-Seltzer (in addition to price) is its sodium content. Those on salt-restricted diets should limit their sodium intake, and anyone with hypertension, diabetes, glaucoma, or any other risk factors for heart disease or stroke should consult a physician before taking drugs high in sodium.

Combinations. See the discussion beginning on page 138.

One final note: Aspirin can go bad. The tip-off is a strong odor of vinegar. If you detect this odor, discard the aspirin.

ACETAMINOPHEN

Aspirin may be the pain reliever doctors recommend most, but the leading brand of acetaminophen, Tylenol, is the one Americans currently *use* most. Introduced in the U.S. in 1955, acetaminophen became popular in the 1970s and today accounts for almost 40 percent of the over-the-counter analgesic market, largely because it causes less stomach upset than either aspirin or ibuprofen. In addition to Tylenol, brands include: Allerest Headache Strength, Anacin-3 (all forms), Bromo-Seltzer, Datril, Excedrin P.M., Panadol (all forms), and St. Joseph Aspirin-Free, among others.

Acetaminophen has neither aspirin's preventive medical value nor its antiinflammatory action. Yet in adult doses of 325 to 650 mg every four hours, it's an effective fever-reducer and pain-reliever.

Acetaminophen is the drug of choice for fevers in children under 18. For dosage information, see Chapter 10 or product packaging.

Acetaminophen is also the drug to take for the upset stomach, headache, and death-warmed-over feeling of a hangover. Alcohol irritates the stomach, so during "the moaning after" it's best to avoid aspirin and ibuprofen, both of which might aggravate stomach distress.

Like aspirin, acetaminophen taken during colds increases the release (shedding) of cold virus particles. Increased shedding might spread colds more easily, but as of this writing, no increase in cold transmission has been shown. One study suggests that acetaminophen (and aspirin) cause more nasal cold symptoms than ibuprofen (see Chapter 6).

Tylenol commercials harp on gentleness and claim that Extra-Strength Tylenol is the pain reliever "hospitals use most." Perhaps, but acetaminophen is not completely innocuous. Authorities urge consumers to limit usage to no more than 4,000 mg a day (six extra-strength tablets). At higher doses, it causes side effects, which, unfortunately, have received very little publicity. Doses of more than 5,000 mg per day over several weeks have been shown to cause liver damage, which is aggravated by alcohol. Most of those who develop acetaminophen liver toxicity are alcoholics, but sensitive individuals can suffer liver damage from the drug alone.

At very high doses—above 10,000 mg for adults, lower for children—acetaminophen is also poisonous. Initial symptoms include: stomach distress, nausea, vomiting, loss of appetite, and sweating. Then come three to five days of apparent improvement, after which tenderness or pain develop in the upper-right quadrant of the abdomen (the liver), followed by jaundice, with possible kidney and heart damage, and sometimes death. If you suspect acetaminophen poisoning, call 911. The operator will tell you to take the victim to an emergency medical facility, or instruct you to give syrup of ipecac to induce vomiting. Never give ipecac unless a 911 operator or medical professional recommends it. As mentioned earlier, every home medicine cabinet should contain ipecac. Activated charcoal also helps treat acetaminophen poisoning.

In asthmatics, acetaminophen may trigger asthma attacks, but this occurs much less frequently than it does with aspirin. Those with asthma should consult a physician or pharmacist about the advisability of using this drug.

Pregnant women should ideally avoid all medications, but for fever and pain relief, most physicians recommend acetaminophen over aspirin or ibuprofen. Pregnant women should consult their medical care provider before taking any medication.

High doses of acetaminophen may also cause kidney damage. If you have kidney disease, ask a physician or pharmacist about the advisability of using it.

Acetaminophen rarely causes stomach upset, so there's no reason to market a buffered version. But that's exactly what Bromo-Seltzer is—acetaminophen and sodium bicarbonate, an antacid. The presence of sodium puts Bromo-Seltzer off limits to anyone with hypertension or on a salt-restricted diet. Those with glaucoma, diabetes, or any other risk factors for heart disease or stroke should consult a physician or pharmacist about the advisability of using this product.

IBUPROFEN

Ibuprofen was introduced in 1974 as the prescription drug Motrin, and quickly became popular with women for relief of menstrual cramping. Ten years later, it was deregulated, and now accounts for about 20 percent of the market under such brand names as: Advil, Nuprin, Medipren, Midol, and Trendar.

Like aspirin, ibuprofen's interference with cyclooxygenase inhibits thromboxane-A_2 synthesis, so at first glance it might appear to have the same value in preventing heart attack and stroke. Aspirin's effect, however, is *irreversible,* while ibuprofen's is quickly *reversible.* This detail makes a world of difference in the body. Ibuprofen has no preventive value against the conditions discussed in Chapters 1 through 6. In large doses (600 to 1,800 mg per day) ibuprofen inhibits platelet aggregation and prolongs bleeding time, but unlike aspirin, which prolongs bleeding for up to a week after ingestion of a single dose, ibuprofen's effect reverses within 24 hours, so it carries less risk of bleeding side effects.

Milligram for milligram, ibuprofen is the more potent pain reliever. The relief it provides also lasts longer. A 100 mg dose of ibuprofen provides about as much pain relief as one standard 325 mg tablet of aspirin; and while aspirin lasts about four hours, ibuprofen lasts up to six. The standard pain-relieving dose of ibuprofen is 200 to 400 mg every four to six hours, with a limit of 1,200 mg per day. The higher the dose, the greater the pain relief up to 400 mg. Beyond that, studies show no additional benefit. The antiinflammatory dose is 300 to 600 mg every four to six hours, with a daily limit of 2,400 mg.

Ibuprofen is particularly effective for menstrual cramps (primary dysmenorrhea), which affects an estimated 50 percent of reproductive-age women. Several studies have shown it "clearly superior" to aspirin. The recommended dose is 400 to 800 mg initially, then up to 400 mg four times a day while cramping, backache, malaise, and other symptoms persist.

Other studies have shown 400 mg of ibuprofen to be superior to aspirin (650 mg), and even codeine (60 mg) for treatment of pain following dental surgery. (In addition, aspirin would not be advised because it causes the greatest prolongation of postsurgical bleeding.)

Ibuprofen overdose is possible but rare. Those at greatest risk are the elderly and children under three.

Like aspirin, ibuprofen may cause stomach upset and gastrointestinal bleeding, but it carries less risk of GI side effects and doses of up to 1,200 mg per day produce little, if any, GI bleeding.

Although ibuprofen prolongs bleeding for only a short time, people with clotting disorders or those taking anticoagulants should consult a physician or pharmacist about the advisability of taking ibuprofen and anticoagulants at the same time.

Like aspirin, ibuprofen taken during colds increases viral shedding, which might spread colds more easily, but as of this writing, no increase in cold transmission has been shown. One recent study shows that compared with aspirin and acetaminophen, ibuprofen, when taken for colds, causes less nasal congestion and runny nose.

Ibuprofen may interfere with kidney function and cause sodium and water retention. Those with kidney disease, hypertension, diabetes, glaucoma, congestive heart failure, or a history of heart attack, TIAs, or stroke should consult a physician or pharmacist about the advisability of using it.

Those with a history of hives, asthma, and aspirin sensitivity should also consult a medical professional about using ibuprofen. Like aspirin, it can cause hives, asthma attacks, and on occasion, anaphylaxis. Those who are sensitive to aspirin are often sensitive to ibuprofen as well.

Those with systemic lupus erythematosus should not take ibuprofen. Severe reactions are possible.

Ibuprofen is a nonsteroidal antiinflammatory drug (NSAID). Anyone taking another NSAID should consult a physician or pharmacist about the advisability of taking ibuprofen at the same time.

Pregnant women should not take ibuprofen unless their medical care provider recommends it. Nursing mothers may take up to 2,400 mg a day. There is no measurable excretion of the drug into breast milk.

COMBINATIONS

For relief of fever and pain, drug makers market two combinations: aspirin-caffeine, and aspirin-acetaminophen-caffeine.

Aspirin-caffeine. Products include: Anacin, Midol (some forms), and BC Tablet and Powder. These products all contain about 32 mg of caffeine, approximately one-quarter the amount in a cup of brewed coffee. During the 1970s, American Medical Association investigators found "no evidence" that such a small dose of caffeine adds anything to plain aspirin's effectiveness—except a higher price.

But three recent studies—of headache, sore throat, and postoperative oral surgery pain—show that combinations of aspirin plus 64 mg of caffeine, the amount in two tablets of combination products, provided "significantly greater pain relief" than either plain aspirin or acetaminophen. To see if a little caffeine gives you added pain relief, you might try

Anacin, Midol, and BC. Or take aspirin with a cup of coffee or tea, or a glass of a caffeinated cola.

Aspirin-acetaminophen-caffeine. Products include: Excedrin Extra Strength, Trigesic, and Vanquish, among others. These three-drug combinations typically contain about 200 mg of aspirin, 200 mg of acetaminophen, and 30 mg of caffeine, except Excedrin, which contains 65 mg. The American Pharmaceutical Association recommends against aspirin-acetaminophen combinations because the benefits appear inconsequential while the possible risks have not been adequately evaluated. On the other hand, these products are FDA approved, so the agency is satisfied that they are reasonably safe. If you're inclined to try an aspirin-acetaminophen combination, it might provide greater pain relief than either drug by itself. Instead of buying a combination product, it would be more economical to take generic low-dose aspirin and acetaminophen at the same time with a cup of coffee or tea, or a glass of a caffeinated cola.

CHAPTER TEN

ASPIRIN AND CHILDREN: PARENTS BEWARE

Thirty years ago, parents gave their young children baby aspirin, and commercials for St. Joseph Aspirin for Children were as familiar on black-and-white television as the "Mickey Mouse Club." But during the early 1980s, several studies linked aspirin treatment of certain childhood fevers with development of Reye's syndrome, a potentially fatal disease. Reye's syndrome was associated only with aspirin treatment of children's colds, flu, and chickenpox. It's often difficult, however, for parents to tell what's causing a child's fever. To play it safe, most parents stopped treating *all* childhood fevers with aspirin, and many stopped giving aspirin for any reason. Today, acetaminophen is overwhelmingly the drug of choice for childhood fever and pain.

DR. KAPILA AND DR. REYE

C.C. Kapila, a physician in southern India in the 1950s, suffered the same fate as Lawrence Craven—only worse. Thirty years after Craven proposed that aspirin might prevent heart attack, his contribution to preventive medicine has been belatedly recognized. Kapila has not been as fortunate. Five years before Dr. Ralph Douglas Kenneth Reye identified "Reye's syndrome," Kapila named the identical condition "Kapila disease." In 1975, in a brief report on Reye's syndrome in the *Journal of the American Medical Association,* researchers at Milwaukee Children's Hospital made a feeble attempt to rename the disease Kapila-Reye's syndrome—but to no avail. Reye's work is remembered fondly; Kapila's has been largely forgotten.

Kapila's discovery came about when he examined the medical records of 9,459 Indian children who contracted influenza A, the most severe flu, during the winter of 1957–58. Thirty (0.3 percent) developed the same group of serious, sometimes fatal, disorders of the central nervous system and liver. Kapila and his colleagues published their findings in the *British Medical Journal* in 1958. Oddly, this article in a prestigious medical journal made little impression. Five years later in 1963, Reye (1912–77), a pathologist in Sydney, Australia, published his report in another British journal, *The Lancet.* From 1951 through 1962, he identified 21 cases of a strange disorder involving brain and liver damage in Australian children.

Within a few years of Reye's article, case reports of Reye's syndrome were appearing regularly in medical journals. In 1977, the federal Centers for Disease Control (CDC) in Atlanta deemed it prevalent and serious enough to warrant a national surveillance program. From 1977 through 1982, the CDC reported an average of about 250 cases a year, with a death rate of about 25 percent. An estimated 4,000 cases of Reye's syndrome have been reported in the U.S. since 1970.

Typically, Reye's syndrome develops in children who appear to be recovering uneventfully from colds, flu, or chickenpox. Then suddenly they develop persistent vomiting, followed by lethargy, disorientation, hostility, inability to recognize family members, and twitching movements. Within a few days, children who do not improve fall into a coma and die. On autopsy, they show serious liver degeneration.

The cause of Reye's syndrome was a mystery until 1982 when three studies all linked it with aspirin treatment of viral illnesses:

• Researchers from the CDC compared the medical histories of 25 Michigan children with Reye's syndrome with similar children who did not develop the disease (matched controls). The only significant difference was the use of aspirin to treat the Reye's children's winter colds and flu. "Although Reye's syndrome can develop in the absence of aspirin ingestion," the researchers wrote in the *Journal of the American Medical Association,* "our data indicate that aspirin taken during viral illness may contribute to its development."

• Ohio Department of Health investigators compared 97 cases of Reye's syndrome in that state's children with matched controls. Again, the only significant difference was that the affected children had been given aspirin for viral infections.

• And Arizona researchers came to the same conclusion about 19 Reye's syndrome cases they studied.

Accompanying the Arizona report, the journal *Pediatrics* ran two contradictory editorials. One urged "a total community effort" to dissuade parents from treating childhood viral fevers with aspirin: "Each of these studies is individually statistically significant. Considering them together, their significance is enormous. There is no reasonable likelihood that these results are a consequence of chance alone.'' The other dismissed the three studies as methodologically flawed.

To settle the issue, the U.S. Public Health Service did a rigorous study, which in 1985 confirmed the aspirin-Reye's connection. Since then, physicians have strongly discouraged giving aspirin to children suffering viral infections, and many discourage aspirin treatment of all childhood fevers. Reye's syndrome is rare in children over 16, but many physicians urge parents to treat fevers with acetaminophen until children are 18.

As fewer and fewer parents have given their feverish children aspirin, the number of Reye's syndrome cases has plummeted. In 1982, when the aspirin-Reye connection was first established, 213 cases were reported. In 1989, there were just 27.

Reye's syndrome is extremely rare in adults, but in the U.S., at least 25 have developed it. If you're concerned, take acetaminophen for fever.

Recently, Reye's syndrome has been diagnosed on autopsy in a few adults who died of AIDS. As this book goes to press, aspirin's role, if any, remains unclear.

CHILDHOOD "OWIES" AND ASPIRIN

Because acetaminophen has become the drug of choice for childhood fever, many parents also give it automatically for everyday bumps, scrapes, cuts, and other minor injuries. This is fine, but assuming the child appears healthy and has a normal temperature, there's no reason not to give baby aspirin— except that it may be hard to find. The standard children's aspirin tablet contains 81 mg, one-quarter the standard adult dose. Children's aspirin packaging contains dosage information, but here's what the American Pharmaceutical Association recommends:

Child's Age	Number of 81 mg doses every four hours	Maximum total dose in 24 hours (in mg)
Under 2	Consult the child's physician	—
2–4	2 (162 mg)	800
4–6	3 (243 mg)	1,200
6–9	4 (324 mg)	1,600
9–11	5 (405 mg)	2,000
11–12	6 (486 mg)	2,400

No child should be given a nonprescription pain reliever regularly for more than three days without consulting a physician. When in doubt about how much aspirin—or any drug—to give a child, consult your physician or pharmacist.

THE RETURN OF BABY ASPIRIN—FOR ADULTS

Due to concern about Reye's syndrome during the 1980s, parents stampeded away from acetylsalicylic acid, and baby aspirin sales plummeted. In 1988, Plough pharmaceutical company of Memphis, Tennessee, stopped making St. Joseph Aspirin for Children. (The company now markets an acetaminophen product, St. Joseph Aspirin-Free Fever Reducer for Children.)

At the same time, aspirin's role in the prevention of heart attack and stroke was becoming established, and at 81 mg per pill, baby aspirin turned out to be a convenient way to take the low doses some doctors were beginning to recommend for their prevention. Now many physicians advise those at risk for heart attack, stroke, colon cancer, and the other conditions discussed in Chapters 1 through 6 to take baby aspirin instead of the standard 325 mg pills. Only it's not called "baby aspirin" anymore: Plough has resurrected its old standby as St. Joseph Adult Aspirin Low Strength.

CHAPTER ELEVEN

SHOULD *YOU* TAKE ASPIRIN REGULARLY? AND IF SO, HOW MUCH?

No doubt about it: Aspirin is miraculous, quite possibly the most cost-effective preventive medicine of all time. But despite its over-the-counter availability, it's also potentially hazardous, and some people should not take it—even at low preventive doses. If you believe that aspirin might contribute to your well-being, consider the questions in this chapter, and then discuss the answers—and your specific medical situation—with your doctor. Even if it appears that aspirin would do you no harm, your doctor may be aware of important aspects of your medical history that might preclude your using it. In addition, your physician may be *unaware* of some of aspirin's new uses and side effects. Take this book along when you visit your doctor so that he or she can read the section(s) that apply to you and check the relevant references.

Are You at Risk for Heart Disease?

• Have you ever had a heart attack, angina attack, arrhythmia, congestive heart failure, rheumatic heart disease, or any other heart or arterial problem? If so, your physician might encourage you to take low-dose aspirin regularly.

• Have any of your blood relatives—mother, father, sisters, brothers, children, grandparents, or blood-related aunts and uncles—had a heart attack, angina, congestive heart failure, angioplasty, coronary artery bypass surgery, or cardiac arrhythmias? Have any of your relatives died of heart disease? The more heart disease in your family, the greater your risk.

• How old are you? After about age 40, the older you are, the more likely your physician is to recommend regular low-dose aspirin.

• Do you have diabetes? More than 80 percent of diabetics die of cardiovascular diseases. In reports to date, regular low-dose aspirin has been shown to be safe for those with diabetic retinopathy. Increasingly, physicians recommend regular low-dose aspirin for diabetics.

• Do you smoke? Or have you quit recently? Smoking increases risk of cardiovascular diseases. If you smoke, quit. In addition, physicians increasingly recommend low-dose aspirin for smokers and ex-smokers.

• Do you have high blood pressure? If so, it should be reduced by life-style modifications and possibly with medication. In addition, physicians increasingly recommend low-dose aspirin for those with hypertension.

• Do you have elevated cholesterol? High cholesterol should be reduced by increasing exercise, adopting a low-fat diet, and possibly with the help of medication. In addition, physicians increasingly recommend low-dose aspirin for those with significantly elevated cholesterol.

• Are you significantly overweight? Those who are clinically obese—20 percent over recommended weight—should lose those extra pounds through a combination of regular moderate exercise, a low-fat diet, and possibly professional help. In addition, physicians increasingly recommend low-dose aspirin.

• Do you usually feel time-pressured and impatient, especially in lines? If so, you may have a Type-A personality. Counseling might help you relax. In addition, physicians increasingly recommend regular low-dose aspirin for Type-A's.

• Do you take birth control pills? If so, and you're over 35 and have any of the risk factors mentioned above, review your contraceptive choice with your family planning provider. In addition, your physician might recommend low-dose aspirin.

Are You at Risk for Stroke?

• Risk factors for stroke are similar to those for heart disease. High blood pressure is particularly important; family history, age, diabetes, smoking, and cholesterol also play a role. In addition:

• Have you had a prior stroke or transient ischemic attack (TIA)? If so, your physician might recommend low-dose aspirin.

• Do you have a carotid bruit? Abnormalities in the carotid artery increase stroke risk. Your physician might recommend low-dose aspirin.

• Are you African American? If so, you may be at risk for stroke, and your physician might recommend low-dose aspirin.

Are You at Risk for Any Other Thrombotic Condition?

• Do you have peripheral artery disease, intermittent claudication, chronically swollen ankles, or thrombophlebitis? If so, your physician might recommend low-dose aspirin.

Are You at Risk for Colorectal Cancer?

• Has anyone in your family ever had colorectal cancer? Do colon polyps run in your family? If so, your physician might recommend low-dose aspirin.
• How old are you? After about age 50, the older you are, the more likely your physician is to recommend low-dose aspirin.
• Do you have colitis? If so, you may be at increased risk for this cancer, and your physician might recommend low-dose aspirin.
• Do you eat a high-fat, low-fiber diet? If so, you may be at risk for colorectal cancer. The American Cancer Society recommends evolving your diet to one lower in fat and higher in fiber by eating more whole grains and fresh fruits and vegetables. In addition, your physician might recommend low-dose aspirin.
• Are you African American? African Americans have a somewhat increased rate of colorectal cancer. Your physician might recommend low-dose aspirin.

Are You Pregnant or Trying to Conceive?

• In general, pregnant women should not take aspirin (or any medication) unless a physician recommends it. If you are at risk for pregnancy-induced hypertension, umbilical placental insufficiency, or if you have lupus anticoagulant autoantibodies, low-dose aspirin might help. Consult your doctor or prenatal care provider.

Do You Have Migraine Headaches?

• Some studies (see References for Chapter 6) suggest that low-dose aspirin might help prevent them. Discuss them with your physician.

Are You at Risk for Cataracts?

• Risk factors include: a family history, smoking, diabetes, nearsightedness, certain eye injuries, corticosteroid drug use, and exposure to radiation. Some studies (see References for Chapter 6) suggest that low-dose aspirin might help prevent cataracts. Discuss them with your physician.

Do You Have Diabetic Retinopathy?

• As this book goes to press, only two studies have been published, and only one shows any preventive value for low-dose aspirin. These studies are cited in the References for Chapter 6. Discuss them with your physician.

Do You Have Insomnia, a Weight Problem, or Wheat Intolerance?

• The evidence is sketchy, but a few studies and case reports (see References for Chapter 6) suggest that aspirin might help. Discuss them with your physician.

Is There a Hip Replacement in Your Future?

• Aspirin taken around the time of surgery may help prevent complications. The one study is cited in the References for Chapter 6. Discuss it with your physician.

Does Aspirin Upset Your Stomach?

• As discussed in Chapter 9, there are several ways to prevent aspirin-induced stomach distress. If aspirin upsets your stomach, discuss this side effect with your physician.

Do You Have Any Bleeding Problems?

• If you bruise easily, develop frequent red spots in the whites of your eyes, take any anticoagulant medication, anticipate surgery, have a vitamin K deficiency, or have hemophilia, von Willebrand's disease, or any other clotting disorder, your physician might advise you against using aspirin regularly, and possibly at all.

Do You Have a Gastrointestinal Illness?

• If you have ulcers, iron-deficiency anemia, or GI problems related to alcoholism, you may not be able to tolerate aspirin, even at low, preventive doses. Discuss your condition with your physician.

Do You Have a Hearing Problem?

• Therapeutic doses of aspirin may cause ringing in the ears (tinnitus). If you have tinnitus or any hearing problem, ask your physician about the advisability of taking aspirin.

Do You Have Asthma or Hives?

• If so, you may be sensitive to aspirin. Discuss your situation with your physician.
• If you are aspirin-sensitive, desensitization is possible. Consult your physician.

Do You Have Gout?

• Aspirin may trigger gout attacks. If you have it, ask your physician about the advisability of taking aspirin.

Do You Have Macular Degeneration?

• As this book goes to press, low-dose aspirin has not been linked to aggravation of macular degeneration. But if you have this form of vision impairment, ask your physician about the advisability of taking aspirin.

Do You Take Vitamin C, Folic Acid, or Iron Regularly?

• Aspirin may interfere with their absorption. Discuss your situation with your physician or with a registered dietitian.

Do You Take Any Other Drugs Regularly?

• Aspirin interacts with many other drugs. Check the list in Chapter 8. If you take any listed medication, ask your physician about the advisability of taking aspirin.

HOW MUCH ASPIRIN SHOULD YOU TAKE?

If your physician says you might benefit from regular low-dose aspirin, the next question is: How much? The latest research shows that a daily dose as low as 30 mg has significant stroke-preventive value. This action depends on the same mechanism that makes aspirin useful in prevention of heart attack, namely, inhibition of cyclooxygenase, which prevents the formation of thromboxane-A_2 and reduces the likelihood of thrombosis. Is 30 mg a day sufficient to prevent heart attack? Maybe, but maybe not.

In the aspirin–heart attack studies discussed in Chapter 1, researchers used doses ranging from 324 mg every other day to 1,500 mg a day. But to date there have been only a few studies of the optimal dose for cyclooxygenase-thromboxane inhibition:

- A 1985 report by Italian researchers suggested that 20 mg of aspirin largely inhibited thromboxane, but not entirely.
- A 1989 investigation by German scientists compared 30 mg a day with 1,000 mg a day for prevention of second heart attacks. After two years of follow-up, the low dose was as effective as the higher one.
- Another 1989 study by another German group compared several doses of aspirin: 20 mg twice a day, 40 mg once a day, 80 mg every other day, and 324 mg (one standard tablet) once a day. The 324 mg dose produced the best platelet suppression, with 80 mg every other day being almost as effective, and the other regimens significantly less so. The researchers concluded that the best low dose for heart attack prevention was somewhere between the 324 mg given every other day in the Physicians' Health Study (the equivalent of 162 mg a day), and one standard 324 mg aspirin tablet a day. (The equivalent of approximately one-half an aspirin a day also had the greatest effect in preventing deaths from colorectal cancer.)

Based on these studies, the best low dose of aspirin would appear to fall somewhere between a daily 162 and 324 mg. Of course, no dose provides any benefit unless you take it regularly. To use aspirin regularly, it must fit conveniently into your life. Some people have no problem taking a pill every other day, but that's confusing for those who prefer to take medicine daily. Some have no problem cutting pills into pieces, but others would rather be spared the hassle. As a result, physicians currently make a variety of recommendations. The most popular are:

- One 81 mg adult low-strength aspirin tablet a day
- Two 81 mg adult low-strength aspirin tablets a day
- Half a standard aspirin tablet (162 mg) a day
- One standard aspirin (324 mg) a day

- One standard aspirin every other day (the equivalent of 162 mg a day)

Ask your physician how much aspirin you should take, and how often.

As this book goes to press, some evidence suggests that those who stop taking low-dose aspirin regularly experience a sudden increase (rebound) in thromboxane levels and platelet stickiness, which might increase risk of heart attack, stroke, and other aspirin-prevented conditions. If your doctor suggests you take low-dose aspirin regularly, and you'd like to stop for any reason, discuss your intention with your physician before you do so.

NOT BY ASPIRIN ALONE

Remember, even if your physician encourages you to take aspirin regularly, it's *no substitute* for risk-factor reduction: quitting smoking, losing weight, eating a low-fat diet, enjoying regular moderate exercise, and controlling blood pressure, cholesterol, and stress. Aspirin may be miraculous, but it works best for those who take good care of themselves.

References

Chapter One
ASPIRIN HELPS PREVENT AND TREAT HEART ATTACK AND ANGINA

Altman, L. K. "Little-Known Doctor Who Found New Use for Common Aspirin." *New York Times*, July 9, 1991, B6.

Anon (editorial). "Aspirin After Myocardial Infarction," *The Lancet* (1980) 8179:1172.

Aspirin Myocardial Infarction Study Research Group. "Aspirin and Myocardial Infarction: A New National Cooperative Trial," *Journal of the American Medical Association* (1975) 232:1359.

————. "A Randomized, Controlled Trial of Aspirin in Persons Recovered from Myocardial Infarction," *Journal of the American Medical Association* (1980) 243:661.

Basinski, A., and C. D. Naylor. "Aspirin and Fibrinolysis in Acute Myocardial Infarction: Meta-Analytic Evidence for Synergy," *Journal of Clinical Epidemiology* (1991) 44:1085.

Becker, R. C. "Aspirin in Acute MI and Angioplasty," *Choices in Cardiology/Family Practitioner Series* (1992) 1:1:8.

Boston Collaborative Drug Surveillance Group. "Regular Aspirin Intake and Myocardial Infarction," *British Medical Journal* (1974) 1:440.

Breddin, K., et al. "Secondary Prevention of Myocardial Infarction: A Comparison of Acetylsalicylic Acid, Placebo, and Phenprocoumon," *Haemostasis* (1980) 9:325.

Cairns, J. A., et al. "Aspirin, Sulfinpyrazone, or Both in Unstable Angina," *New England Journal of Medicine* (1985) 313:1369.

Carpenter, A. L., and J. C. Caravalho, Jr. "Early Public Use of Aspirin in the Face of Probable Ischemic Chest Pain," *The Lancet* (1990) 8682:163.

Coronary Drug Project Research Group. "Aspirin in Coronary Heart Disease," *Journal of Chronic Disease* (1976) 29:625.

Craven, L. L. "Acetylsalicylic Acid: Possible Preventive of Coronary Thrombosis," *Annals of Western Medicine and Surgery* (1950) 4:95.

———. "Experiences with Aspirin in the Nonspecific Prophylaxis of Coronary Thrombosis," *Mississippi Valley Medical Journal* (1953) 75:38.

———. "Prevention of Coronary and Cerebral Thrombosis," *Mississippi Valley Medical Journal* (1956) 78:213.

Dalen, J. E. "An Apple a Day, or an Aspirin a Day?," *Archives of Internal Medicine* (1991) 151:1066.

Das, B. N., and V. S. Banka. "Coronary Artery Disease in Women: How It Is—and Isn't—Unique," *Postgraduate Medicine* (1992) 91:4:197.

Davis, R. F., and E. G. Engleman. "Incidence of Myocardial Infarction in Patients with Rheumatoid Arthritis," *Arthritis and Rheumatism* (1974) 17:527.

Elwood, P. C., et al. "A Randomized Controlled Trial of Acetylsalicylic Acid in the Secondary Prevention of Mortality from Myocardial Infarction," *British Medical Journal* (1974) 1:436.

Elwood, P. C., et al. "Aspirin and Secondary Mortality After Myocardial Infarction," *The Lancet* (1979) 8156:1314.

Elwood, P. C., and W. O. Williams. "A Randomized Controlled Trial of Aspirin in the Prevention of Early Mortality in Myocardial Infarction," *Journal of the Royal College of General Practitioners* (1979) 29:413.

Ernst, E., et al. "Garlic and Blood Lipids," *British Medical Journal* (1985) 291:139.

Gavaghan, T. P., et al. "Immediate Postoperative Aspirin Improves Vein Graft Patency Early and Late After Coronary Artery Bypass Surgery: A Placebo-Controlled, Randomized Study," *Circulation* (1991) 83:1526.

Heikinheimo, R., and K. Jarvinen. "Acetylsalicylic Acid and Arteriosclerotic-Thromboembolic Diseases in the Aged," *Journal of the American Geriatric Society* (1971) 19:403.

ISIS-2 Collaborative Group. "Randomized Trial of Intravenous Streptokinase, Oral Aspirin, Both, or Neither Among 17,187 Cases of Suspected Acute Myocardial Infarction: ISIS-2," *The Lancet* (1988) 8607:349.

ISIS-3 Collaborative Group. "ISIS-3: A Randomized Comparison of Streptokinase, vs. Tissue Plasminogen Activator vs. Antistreplase and of Aspirin Plus Heparin vs. Aspirin Alone Among 41,299 Cases of Suspected Acute Myocardial Infarction," *The Lancet* (1992) 339:753.

Kingsley, C. M., and C. G. Satyendra. "How to Reduce the Risk of Coronary Artery Disease," *Postgraduate Medicine* (1992) 91:4:147.

Lavie, C. J., et al. "Exercise and the Heart: Good, Benign, or Evil?," *Postgraduate Medicine* (1992) 9:2:130.

Lewis, D. H., et al. "Protective Effects of Aspirin Against Acute Myocardial Infarction and Death in Men with Unstable Angina," *New England Journal of Medicine* (1983) 309:396.

Mahon, J., et al. "Use of Acetylsalicylic Acid by Physicians and in the Community," *Journal of the Canadian Medical Association* (1991) 145:1107.

Manson, J. E., et al. "A Prospective Study of Aspirin Use and Primary Prevention of Cardiovascular Disease in Women," *Journal of the American Medical Association* (1991) 266:521.

Mustard, J. F., et al. "Aspirin in the Treatment of Cardiovascular Disease: A Review," *American Journal of Medicine* (1983) 75(Suppl.):43.

Overmyer, R. H. "Improving the Chances for Post-MI Reperfusion with Thrombolytics," *Modern Medicine* (1992) 60:1:86.

Persantine-Aspirin Reinfarction Study Research Group. "The Persantine-Aspirin Reinfarction Study," *Circulation* (1980) 62:Suppl V:V–85.

Peto, R., et al. "Randomized Trial of Prophylactic Daily Aspirin in British Male Physicians," *British Medical Journal* (1988) 296:313.

Ridker, P. M., et al. "Low-Dose Aspirin Therapy for Chronic Stable Angina: A Randomized, Placebo-Controlled Trial," *Annals of Internal Medicine* (1991) 114:835.

Ritter, J. M. "Placebo-Controlled, Double-Blind Clinical Trials Can Impede Medical Progress," *The Lancet* (1980) 8178:1126.

Roberts, H. R., and J. N. Lozier. "New Perspectives on the Coagulation Cascade," *Hospital Practice* (1992) 27:1:97.

Satler, L. F., and C. E. Rackley. "Update on Unstable Angina," *Hospital Medicine* (1992) 28:2:33.

Schwartz, L., et al. "Aspirin and Dipyridamole in the Prevention of Restenosis After Percutaenous Transluminal Coronary Angioplasty," *New England Journal of Medicine* (1988) 318:1714.

Spranger, M., et al. "Sex Differences in the Antithrombotic Effect of Aspirin," *Stroke* (1989) 20:34.

Steering Committee of the Physicians' Health Study Research Group. "Preliminary Report: Findings from the Aspirin Component of the Ongoing Physicians' Health Study," *New England Journal of Medicine* (1988) 320:262.

———. "Final Report on the Aspirin Component of the Ongoing Physicians' Health Study," *New England Journal of Medicine* (1989) 321:129.

Taylor, R. R., et al. "Effects of Low-Dose Aspirin on Restenosis After Coronary Angioplasty," *American Journal of Cardiology* (1991) 68:874.

Théroux, P., et al. "Aspirin, Heparin, or Both to Treat Acute Unstable Angina," *New England Journal of Medicine* (1988) 319:1105.

Vetrovec, G. W., et al. "Intracoronary Thrombus in Syndromes of Unstable Angina," *American Heart Journal* (1981) 102:1202.

Wallentin, L. C., et al. "Aspirin After an Episode of Unstable Coronary Artery Disease: Long-Term Effects on the Risk for Myocardial Infarction, Occurrence of Severe Angina, and the Need for Revascularization," *Journal of the American College of Cardiology* (1991) 18:1587.

Weiss, H. J., and L. M. Aledort. "Impaired Platelet/Connective Tissue Reaction in Man After Aspirin Ingestion," *The Lancet* (1967) 7514:495.

Weiss, H. J., et al. "The Effect of Salicylates on the Hemostatic Properties of Platelets in Man," *Journal of Clinical Investigations* (1968) 47:2169.

Whelan, A. M., et al. "The Effect of Aspirin on Niacin-Induced Cutaneous Reactions," *Journal of Family Practice* (1992) 34:165.

Chapter Two
ASPIRIN HELPS PREVENT STROKE AND SENILITY

Antiplatelet Trialists' Collaboration. "Secondary Prevention of Vascular Disease by Prolonged Antiplatelet Treatment," *British Medical Journal* (1988) 296:320.

Atrial Fibrillation Study Group. "Stroke Prevention in the Atrial Fibrillation Study," *Circulation* (1991) 84:527.

Barnett, H. J. M., et al. "Aspirin: Effective in Males Threatened with Stroke," *Stroke* (1978) 9:295.

Bousser, M. G., et al. "AICLA Controlled Trial of Aspirin and Dipyridamole in the Secondary Prevention of Atherothrombotic Cerebral Ischemia," *Stroke* (1983) 14:5.

Brass, L. M., et al. "Transient Ischemic Attacks in the Elderly: Diagnosis and Treatment," *Geriatrics* (1992) 47:5:36.

Bundlie, S. R. "Ischemic Stroke: How to Keep the First One from Happening," *Postgraduate Medicine* (1991) 90:8:56.

Canadian Cooperative Study Group. "A Randomized Trial of Aspirin and Sulfinpyrazone in Threatened Stroke," *New England Journal of Medicine* (1978) 299:53.

Cebul, R. D. "Aspirin and MID: Notes of Caution," *Journal of the American Geriatric Society* (1989) 37:573.

Collins, R., et al. "Blood Pressure, Stroke, Coronary Heart Disease, and Short-Term Reduction in Blood Pressure: An Overview of Randomized Drug Trials in Their Epidemiological Context," *The Lancet* (1990) 8693:827.

Day, H. J. "Stroke Prevention Therapy: Aspirin vs. Ticlopidine," *Drug Therapy* (1992) 22:2:31.

Dutch TIA Trial Study Group. "A Comparison of Two Doses of Aspirin (30 mg vs. 283 mg a day) in Patients After a Transient Ischemic Attack or Minor Stroke," *New England Journal of Medicine* (1991) 325:1261.

Dyken, M. L. "Editorial: Transient Ischemic Attacks and Aspirin, Stroke and Death; Negative Studies and Type II Error," *Stroke* (1983) 14:2.

European Stroke Prevention Study Group. "The European Stroke Prevention Study (ESPS)," *The Lancet* (1987) 8572:1351.

Fields, W. S., et al. "Controlled Trial of Aspirin in Cerebral Ischemia," *Stroke* (1977) 8:301.

Furlan, A. J. "Transient Ischemic Attacks: Recognition and Management," *Heart Disease and Stroke* (1992) 1:1:33.

Haas, W. K. "Aspirin for the Limping Brain," *Stroke* (1977) 8:299.

Harrison, M. J. "Role of Platelets and Antiplatelet Agents in Cerebrovascular Disease: Clues from Trials," *Circulation* (1990) 81(Suppl. I):I20.

Hershey, L. A. "Stroke Prevention in Women: Role of Aspirin vs. Ticlopidine," *American Journal of Medicine* (1991) 91:288.

Koller, R. L. "Prevention of Recurrent Ischemic Stroke," *Postgraduate Medicine* (1991) 90:8:81.

Kutner, M., et al. "Physicians' Attitudes Toward Oral Anticoagulants and Antiplatelet Agents for Stroke Prevention in Elderly Patients with Atrial Fibrillation," *Archives of Internal Medicine* (1991) 151:1950.

Meyer, J. S., et al. "Randomized Clinical Trial of Daily Aspirin Therapy in Multi-Infarct Dementia," *Journal of the American Geriatrics Society* (1989) 37:549.

SALT Collaborative Group. "Swedish Aspirin Low-Dose Trial (SALT) of 75 mg Aspirin as Secondary Prophylaxis After Cerebrovascular Ischemic Events," *The Lancet* (1991) 8779:1345.

Sivenius, J., et al. "The European Stroke Prevention Study: Results According to Sex," *Neurology* (1991) 41:1189.

Sorensen, P. S., et al. "Acetylsalicylic Acid in the Prevention of Stroke in Patients with Reversible Cerebral Ischemic Attacks: A Danish Cooperative Study," *Stroke* (1983) 14:15.

Stachenko, S. J., et al. "Aspirin in Transient Ischemic Attacks and Minor Stroke: A Meta-Analysis," *Family Practice Research Journal* (1991) 11:179.

UK-TIA Study Group. "United Kingdom Transient Ischemic Attack Aspirin Trial: Interim Results," *British Medical Journal* (1988) 296:316.

Wolf, P. A., et al. "Atrial Fibrillation as an Independent Risk Factor for Stroke: The Framingham Study," *Stroke* (1991) 22:983.

Chapter Three
ASPIRIN HELPS PREVENT AND TREAT OTHER SERIOUS CARDIOVASCULAR CONDITIONS

Anon. "Low-Dose Aspirin Found to Slow Peripheral Artery Disease Course," *Family Practice News* (1992) 22:2:1.

Domoto, D. T., et al. "Combined Aspirin and Sulfinpyrazone in the Prevention of Recurrent Hemodialysis Vascular Access Thrombosis," *Thrombosis Research* (1991) 62:737.

Giansante, C., et al. "Treatment of Intermittent Claudication with Antiplatelet Agents," *Journal of Internal Medical Research* (1990) 18:400.

McCardel, B. R., et al. "Aspirin Prophylaxis and Surveillance of Pulmonary Embolism and Deep Vein Thrombosis in Total Hip Arthroplasty," *Journal of Arthroplasty* (1990) 5:181.

Chapter Four
ASPIRIN MAY HELP PREVENT COLON CANCER

Alcorn, J. M. "Colorectal Cancer Prevention: A Primary Care Approach," *Geriatrics* (1992) 47:2:24.

American Cancer Society. "1989 Survey of Physicians' Attitudes and Practices in Early Cancer Detection," *CA Cancer Journal* (1990) 40:2:77.

Baron, J. A., and E. R. Greenberg. "Could Aspirin Really Prevent Colon Cancer?," *New England Journal of Medicine* (1991) 325:1644.

Giovannucci, E., et al. "Relationship of Diet to Risk of Colorectal Adenoma in Men," *Journal of the National Cancer Institute* (1992) 84:91.

Kune, G. A., et al. "Colorectal Cancer, Chronic Illnesses, Operations, and Medications: Case-Control Results from the Melbourne Colorectal Cancer Study," *Cancer Research* (1988) 48:4399.

Labayle, D., et al. "Sulindac Causes Regression of Rectal Polyps in Familial Adenomatous Polyposis," *Gastroenterology* (1991) 101:635.

Lee, M. W. "Colorectal Cancer: Recent Development and Continuing Controversies," *Postgraduate Medicine* (1992) 91:1:153.

Lynch, N. R., et al. "Mechanism of Inhibition of Tumour Growth by Aspirin and Indomethacin," *British Cancer Journal* (1978) 38:503.

Paganini-Hill, A., et al. "Aspirin Use and Chronic Diseases: A Cohort Study of the Elderly," *British Medical Journal* (1989) 299:1247.

Pollard, M., and P. H. Luckert. "Indomethacin Treatment of Rats with Dimethylhydrazine-Induced Intestinal Tumors," *Cancer Treatment Reports* (1980) 64:1323.

Rosenberg, L., et al. "A Hypothesis: Nonsteroidal Anti-Inflammatory Drugs Reduce the Incidence of Large-Bowel Cancer," *Journal of the National Cancer Institute* (1991) 83:355.

Selby, J. V., et al. "A Case-Control Study of Screening Sigmoidoscopy and Mortality from Colorectal Cancer," *New England Journal of Medicine* (1992) 326:653.

Thun, M. J., et al. "Aspirin Use and Reduced Risk of Fatal Colon Cancer," *New England Journal of Medicine* (1991) 325:1593.

Trock, B., et al. "Dietary Fiber, Vegetables, and Colon Cancer: Critical Review and Meta-Analysis of the Epidemiological Evidence," *Journal of the National Institute* (1990) 82:650.

Willett, W. C., et al. "Relation of Meat, Fat, and Fiber Intake to the Risk of Colon Cancer in a Prospective Study Among Women," *New England Journal of Medicine* (1990) 323:1664.

Chapter Five
ASPIRIN AND PREGNANCY: SIGNIFICANT RISKS, MAJOR NEW BENEFITS

Beaufils, M., et al. "Prevention of Preeclampsia by Early Antiplatelet Therapy," *The Lancet* (1985) 8433:840.

Benigni, A., et al. "Effect of Low-Dose Aspirin on Fetal and Maternal Generation of Thromboxane by Platelets in Women at Risk for Pregnancy-Induced Hypertension," *New England Journal of Medicine* (1989) 321:357.

Fitzgerald, D. J., et al. "Decreased Prostacyclin Biosynthesis Preceding the Clinical Manifestation of Pregnancy-Induced Hypertension," *Circulation* (1987) 75:956.

Hertz-Picciotto, I., et al. "The Risks and Benefits of Taking Aspirin During Pregnancy," *Epidemiologic Reviews* (1990) 12:108.

Imperiale, T. F., and A. Stollenwerk-Petrulis. "A Meta-Analysis of Low-Dose Aspirin for the Prevention of Pregnancy-Induced Hypertensive Disease," *Journal of the American Medical Association* (1991) 266:261.

Karboski, J. A. "Medication Selection for Pregnant Women," *Drug Therapy* (1992) 22:2:53.

Masoti, G., et al. "Differential Inhibition of Prostacyclin Production and Platelet Aggregation by Aspirin," *The Lancet* (1979) 8154:1213.

McParland, P., et al. "Doppler Ultrasound and Aspirin in Recognition and Prevention of Pregnancy-Induced Hypertension," *The Lancet* (1990) 335:1552.

Park, C. H. "Etiologic Heterogeneity of Anencephalus and Spina Bifida," *Dissertations Abstracts* (1991) 52/06-B:3019.

Rudolph, A. M. "Effects of Aspirin and Acetaminophen in Pregnancy and in the Newborn," *Archives of Internal Medicine* (1981) 141:358.

Schiff, E., et al. "The Use of Aspirin to Prevent Pregnancy-Induced Hypertension and Lower the Ratio of Thromboxane-A_2 to Prostacyclin in Relatively High-Risk Pregnancies," *New England Journal of Medicine* (1989) 321:351.

Trudinger, B. J., et al. "Low-Dose Aspirin Therapy Improves Fetal Weight in Umbilical Placental Insufficiency," *American Journal of Obstetrics and Gynecology* (1988) 159:681.

Wallenberg, H. C. S., et al. "Low-Dose Aspirin Prevents Pregnancy-Induced Hypertension and Preeclampsia in Angiotensin-Sensitive Primigravidae," *The Lancet* (1986) 8471:1.

Wallenberg, H. C. S., and N. Rotmans. "Prevention of Recurrent Idiopathic Fetal Growth Retardation by Low-Dose Aspirin and Dipyridamole," *American Journal of Obstetrics and Gynecology* (1987) 157:1230.

Walsh, S. W. "Pre-Eclampsia: An Imbalance in Placental Prostacyclin and Thromboxane Production," *American Journal of Obstetrics and Gynecology* (1985) 152:335.

———. "Treatment for the Imbalance of Increased Thromboxane and Decreased Prostacyclin in Preeclampsia," *American Journal of Perinatology* (1989) 6:124.

Werler, M. M., et al. "The Relation of Aspirin Use During the First Trimester of Pregnancy to Congenital Cardiac Defects," *New England Journal of Medicine* (1989) 321:1639.

Chapter Six
THE NEW ASPIRIN FRONTIER

MIGRAINE HEADACHES

Buring, J. E., et al. "Low-Dose Aspirin for Migraine Prophylaxis," *Journal of the American Medical Association* (1990) 264:1711.

Dalessio, D. J. "Migraine, Platelets, and Headache Prophylaxis," *Journal of the American Medical Association* (1978) 239:52.

Grotemeyer, K. H., et al. "Acetylsalicylic Acid vs. Metoprolol in Migraine Prophylaxis: A Double-Blind, Cross-Over Study," *Headache* (1990) 30:639.

O'Neill, B. P., and J. D. Mann. "Aspirin Prophylaxis in Migraine," *The Lancet* (1978) 8101:1179.

Peto, R., et al. "Randomized Trial of Prophylactic Daily Aspirin in British Male Doctors," *British Medical Journal* (1988) 296:313.

CATARACTS

Chew, Y., et al. "Aspirin Effects on the Development of Cataracts in Patients with Diabetes Mellitus," *Archives of Ophthalmology* (1992) 110:339.

Cotlier, E., et al. "Distribution of Salicylate in Lens and Intraocular Fluids and Its Effect on Cataract Formation," *American Journal of Medicine* (1983) 75(Suppl.):83.

Harding, J. J., et al. "Protection Against Cataract by Aspirin, Paracetomol, and Ibuprofen," *Acta Ophthalmologica* (1989) 67:518.

Leske, C. M., et al. "The Lens Opacity Case Control Study: Risk Factors for Cataract," *Archives of Ophthalmology* (1991) 109:244.

Seddon, J. M., et al. "Low-Dose Aspirin and Risk of Cataract in a Randomized Trial of U.S. Physicians," *Archives of Ophthalmology* (1991) 109:252.

Seigel, D., et al. "Aspirin and Cataracts," *Ophthalmology* (1982) 89:47A.

Sharma, Y. R., et al. "Systemic Aspirin and System Vitamin E in Senile Cataracts," *Indian Journal of Ophthalmology* (1989) 37:134.

GALLSTONES

Broomfield, P. H., et al. "Effects of Ursodeoxycholic Acid and Aspirin on the Formation of Lithogenic Bile and Gallstones During Loss of Weight," *New England Journal of Medicine* (1988) 319:1567.

Hood, K., et al. "Prevention of Gallstone Recurrence by Nonsteroidal Anti-Inflammatory Drugs," *The Lancet* (1988) 8622:1223.

Kurata, J. H., et al. "One Gram of Aspirin Per Day Does Not Reduce Risk of Hospitalization for Gallstone Disease," *Digestive Diseases and Sciences* (1991) 36:1110.

Lee, S. P., et al. "Aspirin Prevention of Cholesterol Gallstone Formation in Prairie Dogs," *Science* (1981) 211:1429.

DIABETIC RETINOPATHY

DAMAD Study Group. "Effect of Aspirin Alone and Aspirin Plus Dipyridamole in Early Diabetic Retinopathy: A Multicenter, Randomized, Controlled Clinical Trial," *Diabetes* (1980) 38:491.

Early Treatment Diabetic Retinopathy Study Research Group. "Effects of Aspirin Treatment on Diabetic Retinopathy," *Ophthalmology* (1991) 98:757.

Koneti-Roa, A., et al. "Platelet Coagulant in Diabetes Mellitus: Evidence for Platelet Coagulant Hyperactivity and Platelet Volume," *Journal of Laboratory and Clinical Medicine* (1984) 103:82.

Schachat, A. P. "Can Aspirin Be Used Safely for Patients with Proliferative Diabetic Retinopathy?," *Archives of Ophthalmology* (1992) 110:180.

IMMUNE SYSTEM

Cesario, T. C., et al. "The Regulation of Interferon Production by Aspirin, Other Inhibitors of the Cyclooxygenase Pathway, and Agents Influencing Calcium Channel Flux," *Bulletin of the New York Academy of Sciences* (1989) 65:26.

Graham, N. M, et al. "Adverse Effects of Aspirin, Acetaminophen, and Ibuprofen on Immune Function, Viral Shedding, and Clinical Status in Rhinovirus-Infected Volunteers," *Journal of Infectious Disease* (1990) 162:1277.

Hsia, J., et al. "Immune Modulation by Aspirin During Experimental Rhinovirus Colds," *Bulletin of the New York Academy of Sciences* (1989) 65:45.

Huang, R. T. C., and E. Dietsch. "Anti-Influenza Viral Activity of Aspirin in Cell Culture," *New England Journal of Medicine* (1988) 319:797.

Pottathil, R., et al. "Establishment of the Interferon-Mediated Antiviral State: Role of Fatty Acid Cyclooxygenase," *Proceedings of the National Academy of Sciences* (1980) 77:5437.

INSOMNIA

Houri, P. J., and P. M. Silberfarb. "Effects of Aspirin on the Sleep of Insomniacs," *Current Therapeutic Research* (1980) 28:867.

WEIGHT LOSS

Astrup, A., et al. "Enhanced Thermogenic Responsiveness During Chronic Ephedrine Treatment in Man," *American Journal of Clinical Nutrition* (1985) 42:83.

Horton, T. J., and C. A. Geissler. "Aspirin Potentiates the Effect of Ephedrine on the Thermogenic Response to a Meal in Obese But Not Lean Women," *International Journal of Obesity* (1991) 15:359.

Pasquali, R., et al. "Does Ephedrine Promote Weight Loss in Low-Energy-Adapted Obese Women?," *International Journal of Obesity* (1987) 11:163.

GLUTEN INTOLERANCE

Martin, B. W. "Aspirin for Gluten Enteropathy," *The Lancet* (1982) 8307:1099.

HIP REPLACEMENT COMPLICATIONS

Frieberg, A. A., et al. "The Use of Aspirin to Prevent Heterotopic Ossification After Total Hip Arthroplasty: A Preliminary Report," *Clinical Orthopaedics and Related Research* (1991) 267:93.

LEPROSY

Klenerman, P. "Prostaglandins and Leprosy: A Role for Aspirin?," *Leprosy Review* (1989) 60:51.

Chapter Seven
. . . AND DON'T FORGET ASPIRIN FOR PAIN, FEVER, AND INFLAMMATION

Bland, John H. "The Reversibility of Osteoarthritis: A Review," *American Journal of Medicine* (1983) 75(Suppl.):16.

Csuka, M. E., and D. J. McCarthy. "Aspirin and the Treatment of Rheumatoid Arthritis," *Rheumatic Disease Clinics* (1989) 15:439.

Done, A. K. "The Treatment of Fever: A Review," *American Journal of Medicine* (1983) 75(Suppl.):27.

Lou Harris and Associates. "The Nuprin Pain Report." New York, 1985.

Malmberg, A. B., and T. L. Yaksh. "Hyperalgesia Mediated by Spinal Glutamate or Substance P Receptor Blocked by Spinal Cyclooxygenase Inhibition," *Science* (1992) 257:1276.

Von Witt, R. J. "Topical Aspirin for Wasp Stings," *The Lancet* (1980) 8208/9:1379.

Chapter Eight
ASPIRIN SIDE EFFECTS AND INTERACTIONS

Berstad, K., et al. "Acute Damage of Gastroduodenal Mucosa by Acetylsalicylic Acid: No Prolonged Protection by Antacids," *Alimentary Pharmacology and Therapeutics* (1989) 3:585.

Carson, S. S., et al. "Combined Effects of Aspirin and Noise in Causing Permanent Hearing Loss," *Archives of Otolaryngology* (1989) 115:1070.

Hawkey, C. J., et al. "Prophylaxis of Aspirin-Induced Gastric Mucosal Bleeding with Ranitidine," *Alimentary Pharmacology and Therapeutics* (1988) 2:245.

―――. "Separation of the Impairment of Haemostasis by Aspirin from Mucosal Injury in the Human Stomach," *Clinical Science* (1991) 81:565.

Hawthorne, A. B., et al. "Aspirin-Induced Gastric Mucosal Damage: Prevention by Enteric-Coating and Relation to Prostaglandin Synthesis," *British Journal of Clinical Pharmacology* (1991) 32:77.

Holzer, P., et al. "Intragastric Capsaicin Protects Against Aspirin-Induced Lesion Formation and Bleeding in the Rat Gastric Mucosa," *Gastroenterology* (1989) 96:1425.

Klein, M. L. "Macular Degeneration: Is Aspirin a Risk for Progressive Disease?," *Journal of the American Medical Association* (1991) 266:2279.

Kresel, J. J. "The Epidemiology of Childhood Poisonings: An Investigation into the Methods of Entry Used by Children Under Five Years of Age to Access Children's Aspirin or Chewable Multivitamins," *Dissertation Abstracts* (1981) 50/07-B:2867.

Lanas, A., et al. "Significant Role of Aspirin Use in Patients with Esophagitis," *Journal of Clinical Gastroenterology* (1991) 13:622.

Levy, M. "Aspirin Use in Patients with Major Upper Gastrointestinal Bleeding and Peptic Ulcer Disease," *New England Journal of Medicine* (1974) 290:1158.

Linnoila, M., et al. "Acute Effect of Antipyretic Analgesics, Alone or in Combination with Alcohol, on Human Psychomotor Skills Related to Driving," *British Journal of Clinical Pharmacology* (1974) 1:477.

Makheja, A. N., et al. "Inhibition of Platelet Aggregation and Thromboxane Synthesis by Onion and Garlic," *The Lancet* (1979) 8119:781.

Manning, M. E., and D. D. Stevenson. "Aspirin Sensitivity: A Distressing Reaction That Is Now Often Treatable," *Postgraduate Medicine* (1991) 90:5:227.

Muller, P., et al. "Protection from Gastroduodenal Adverse Effects of Acetylsalicylic Acid with Ranitidine: An Endoscopic Controlled Double-Blind Study of Healthy Volunteers," *Arzneimittelforschung* (1991) 41:638.

Naurang, A. "Risk Factors for Gastrointestinal Ulcers Caused by Nonsteroidal Anti-Inflammatory Drugs," *Journal of Family Practice* (1991) 32:619.

Pawlowicz, A., et al. "Inhalation and Nasal Challenge in the Diagnosis of Aspirin-Induced Asthma," *Allergy* (1991) 46:405.

Roline, R., et al. "Aspirin Increases Blood Alcohol Concentrations in Humans After Ingestion of Ethanol," *Journal of the American Medical Association* (1990) 264:2406.

Settipane, G. A. "Aspirin and Allergic Disease: A Review," *American Journal of Medicine* (1983) 75(Suppl.):102.

Snodgrass, W. R. "Salicylate Toxicity," *Pediatric Clinics of North America* (1986) 33:381.

Stypulkowski, P. H. "Physiological Mechanisms of Salicylate Ototoxicity," *Dissertation Abstracts* (1989) 50/09-B:3860.

Szczeklik, A. "Aspirin-Induced Asthma: New Insights into Pathogenesis and Clinical Presentation of Drug Intolerance," *International Archives of Allergy and Applied Immunology* (1989) 90(Suppl. 1):70.

Thorngren, M., and A. Gustafson. "Effects of Acetylsalicylic Acid and Dietary Intervention on Primary Hemostasis," *American Journal of Medicine* (1983) 75(Suppl.):66.

Truitt, E. B., et al. "Aspirin Attenuation of Alcohol-Induced Flushing and Intoxication in Oriental and Occidental Subjects," *Alcohol* (1987) 22(Suppl. 1):595.

Vertrees, J. E., et al. "Repeated Oral Administration of Activated Charcoal for Treating Aspirin Overdose in Young Children," *Pediatrics* (1990) 85:594.

Weiss, H. J. "Aspirin: A Dangerous Drug?," *Journal of the American Medical Association* (1974) 229:1221.

Williams, W. R., et al. "Aspirin-Like Effects of Selected Food Additives and Industrial Sensitizing Agents," *Clinical and Experimental Allergy* (1989) 19:533.

———. "Aspirin-Sensitive Asthma: Significance of the Cyclooxygenase-Inhibiting and Protein-Binding Properties of Analgesic Drugs," *International Archives of Allergy and Applied Immunology* (1991) 95:303.

Chapter Nine
ASPIRIN VERSUS THE COMPETITION

Chan, W. Y. "Prostaglandins and Nonsteroidal Anti-Inflammatory Drugs in Dysmenorrhea," *Annual Review of Pharmacology and Toxicology* (1983) 23:131.

Forbes, J. A. et al. "An Evaluation of Fluribuprofen, Aspirin, and Placebo in Postoperative Oral Surgery Pain," *Pharmacotherapy* (1989) 9:66.

———. "Evaluation of Ketorolac, Aspirin, and an Acetaminophen-Codeine Combination in Postoperative Oral Surgery Pain," *Pharmacotherapy* (1990) 10:6(Suppl.):77S.

———. "Evaluation of Aspirin, Caffeine, and Their Combinations in Postoperative Oral Surgery Pain," *Pharmacotherapy* (1990) 110:387.

———. "Evaluation of Bromfenac, Aspirin, and Ibuprofen in Postoperative Oral Surgery Pain," *Pharmacotherapy* (1991) 11:64.

Graham, N. M., et al. "Adverse Effects of Aspirin, Acetaminophen, and Ibuprofen on Immune Function, Viral Shedding, and Clinical Status in Rhinovirus-Infected Volunteers," *Journal of Infectious Diseases* (1990) 162:1277.

Hill, J., et al. "A Double-Blind, Crossover Study to Compare Lysine Acetylsalicylic Acid (Aspergesic) with Ibuprofen in the Treatment of Rheumatoid Arthritis," *Journal of Clinical Pharmacy and Therapeutics* (1990) 15:205.

Kumar, S., and D. K. Rex. "Failure of Physicians to Recognize Acetaminophen Hepatotoxicity in Chronic Alcoholics," *Archives of Internal Medicine* (1991) 151:1189.

Laska, E. M., et al. "Caffeine as an Analgesic Adjuvant," *Journal of the American Medical Association* (1984) 251:1711.

Peters, B. H., et al. "Comparison of 650 mg Aspirin and 1000 mg Acetaminophen with Each Other and with Placebo in Moderately Severe Headache," *American Journal of Medicine* (1983) 75(Suppl.):36.

Schachtel, B. P., et al. "Headache Pain Model for Assessing and Comparing the Efficacy of Over-the-Counter Analgesic Agents," *Clinical Pharmacology and Therapeutics* (1991) 50:322.

———. "Caffeine as an Analgesic Adjuvant: A Double-Blind Study Comparing Aspirin with Caffeine to Aspirin and Placebo in Patients with Sore Throat," *Archives of Internal Medicine* (1991) 151:733.

Vanags, D., et al. "The Antiplatelet Effects of Daily Low-Dose Enteric-

Coated Aspirin in Man: A Time Course of Onset and Recovery,''
Thrombosis Research (1991) 59:995.

Chapter Ten
ASPIRIN AND CHILDREN: PARENTS BEWARE

Eagle, B. A., et al. "Reye's Syndrome in an Adult," *Connecticut Medi-cine* (1989) 53:3.

Fulginiti, V. A., et al. "Aspirin and Reye's Syndrome," *Pediatrics* (1982) 69:810.

Hall, S. M. "Reye's Syndrome and Aspirin: A Review," *British Journal of Clinical Practice* (1990) 44:(Suppl. 70):4.

Halpin, J. T., et al. "Reye's Syndrome and Medication Use," *Journal of the American Medical Association* (1982) 248:687.

Hurwitz, E. S. "Reye's Syndrome," *Epidemiologic Reviews* (1989) 11:249.

Jolliet, P., and J. J. Widman. "Reye's Syndrome in Adults with AIDS," *The Lancet* (1990) 335:1457.

Maheady, D. C. "Reye's Syndrome: Review and Update," *Journal of Pediatric Health Care* (1989) 3:246.

Orlowski, J. P. "Reye's Syndrome: A Case-Control Study of Medication Use and Associated Viruses in Australia," *Cleveland Clinic Medical Journal* (1990) 57:323.

Porter, J. D., et al. "Trends in the Incidence of Reye's Syndrome and the Use of Aspirin," *Archives of the Diseases of Children* (1990) 65:826.

Starko, K. M., et al. "Reye Syndrome and Salicylate Use," *Pediatrics* (1980) 66:859.

Tang, T. T., et al. "Reye Syndrome: A Correllated Electron-Microscopic, Viral, and Biochemical Observation," *Journal of the American Medical Association* (1975) 232:13:1339.

Waldman, R. J. "Aspirin as a Risk Factor in Reye's Syndrome," *Journal of the American Medical Association* (1982) 247:3089.

Wilson, J. T., and R. D. Brown. "Reye Syndrome and Aspirin Use: The Role of Prodromal Illness Severity in the Assessment of Relative Risk," *Pediatrics* (1982) 69:822.

Zamula, A. "Reye Syndrome: Decline of a Disease," *FDA Consumer* (1990) November:20.

Chapter Eleven
SHOULD YOU TAKE ASPIRIN REGULARLY? AND IF SO, HOW MUCH?

Anon. "Questions, Concerns Still Bar Wider Use of Aspirin Prophylaxis," *Family Practice News* (1992) 22:8:25.

Dalen, J. E. "An Apple a Day or an Aspirin a Day?," *Archives of Internal Medicine* (1991) 151:1066.

DeGaetano, G., et al. "Pharmacology of Platelet Inhibition in Humans: Implications of the Salicylate-Aspirin Interaction," *Circulation* (1985) 72:1185.

Dutch TIA Trial Study Group. "A Comparison of Two Doses of Aspirin (30 mg vs. 283 mg a day) in Patients After a Transient Ischemic Attack or Minor Stroke," *New England Journal of Medicine* (1991) 325:1261.

Forrester, W., and W. Hoffmann. "Superior Prevention of Reinfarction by 30 mg per Day Aspirin Compared with 1000 mg: Results of a Two-Year Follow-Up Study," *Progress in Clinical and Biological Research* (1989) 301:187.

Lorenz, R. L., et al. "Superior Antiplatelet Action of Alternate Day Pulsed Dosing vs. Split-Dose Administration of Aspirin," *American Journal of Cardiology* (1989) 64:1185.

Patrono, C., et al. "Clinical Pharmacology of Platelet Cyclooxygenase Inhibition," *Circulation* (1985) 72:1177.

Steering Committee of the Physicians' Health Study Research Group. "Final Report on the Aspirin Component of the Ongoing Physicians' Health Study," *New England Journal of Medicine* (1989) 321:129.

Thun, M. J., et al. "Aspirin Use and Reduced Risk of Fatal Colon Cancer," *New England Journal of Medicine* (1991) 325:1593.

Bibliography

American Pharmaceutical Association. *Handbook of Nonprescription Drugs,* 8th ed. Washington, D.C.: American Pharmaceutical Association, 1986.

Amsterdam, Ezra A., and Ann M. Holmes. *Take Care of Your Heart.* New York: Facts on File, 1984.

Consumer Reports. *The Medicine Show.* Mt. Vernon, N.Y.: Consumers Union, 1983.

Cunningham, F. Gary, et al. *Williams Obstetrics,* 18th ed. Norwalk, Conn.: Appleton and Lange, 1989.

Friedman, Meyer, and Diane Ulmer. *Treating Type-A Behavior and Your Heart.* New York: Knopf, 1984.

Ferguson, Tom, M.D. *The No-Nag, No-Guilt, Do-It-Your-Own-Way Guide to Quitting Smoking.* New York: Ballantine, 1989.

Goodman Gilman, Alfred, et al. *Goodman and Gilman's The Pharmacological Basis of Therapeutics,* 7th ed. New York: Macmillan, 1985.

Goor, Ron, M.D., and Nancy Goor. *Eater's Choice: A Food Lover's Guide to Lower Cholesterol.* Boston: Houghton Mifflin, 1992.

Goor, Ron, M.D., Nancy Goor, and Katherine Boyd, R.D. *The Choose to Lose Diet.* Boston: Houghton Mifflin, 1990.

Graedon, Joe, and Teresa Graedon. *The Graedons' Best Medicine.* New York: Bantam, 1991.

Hamilton, Michael, M.D., M.P.H, et al. *The Duke University Medical Center Book of Diet and Fitness.* New York: Fawcett, Columbine, 1990.

Hendler, Sheldon Saul. *The Doctors' Vitamin and Mineral Encyclopedia.* New York: Fireside/Simon and Schuster, 1990.

Holleb, Arthur, ed. *The American Cancer Society Cancer Book.* New York: Doubleday, 1986.

Huff, Barbara, ed. *Physicians' Desk Reference for Nonprescription Drugs 1990.* Oradell, N.J.: Medical Economics Co., 1990.

Kunz, Jeffrey R. M., and Asher J. Finkel, eds. *The American Medical Association Family Medical Guide.* New York: Random House, 1987.

Mann, Charles C., and Mark L. Plummer. *The Aspirin Wars*. New York: Knopf, 1991.

Olin, Bernie R., ed. *Drug Facts and Comparisons*. St. Louis, Mo.: Facts and Comparisons, 1990.

Petrie, Roy H. *Perinatal Pharmacology*. Oradell, N.J.: Medical Economics Books, 1989.

Prevention Magazine. *The Doctors Book of Home Remedies*. Emmaus, Pa.: Rodale Press, 1990.

Renneker, Mark. *Understanding Cancer*. Palo Alto, Calif.: Bull Publishing, 1988.

Rinzler, Carol Ann. *Feed a Cold, Starve a Fever: A Dictionary of Medical Folklore*. New York: Facts on File, 1991.

Simons, Anne, et al. *Before You Call the Doctor*. New York: Ballantine, 1992.

Tarpley, Donald F., et al., eds. *The Columbia University College of Physicians and Surgeons Complete Home Medical Guide*. New York: Crown, 1989.

Wilson, Jean D., et al., eds. *Harrison's Principles of Internal Medicine*, 12th ed. New York: McGraw-Hill, 1991.

Yudofsky, Stuart, et al. *What You Need to Know About Psychiatric Drugs*. New York: Grove Weidenfield, 1991.

Index

10/93 / 10/93

4/97 - 3 ✓ 8/98

THE STANDARD BOOK OF QUILT MAKING AND COLLECTING, Marguerite Ickis. Full information, full-sized patterns for making 46 traditional quilts, also 150 other patterns. Quilted cloths, lame, satin quilts, etc. 483 illustrations. 273pp. 6⅞ x 9⅝. 20582-7 Pa. $4.95

ENCYCLOPEDIA OF VICTORIAN NEEDLEWORK, S. Caulfield, Blanche Saward. Simply inexhaustible gigantic alphabetical coverage of every traditional needlecraft—stitches, materials, methods, tools, types of work; definitions, many projects to be made. 1200 illustrations; double-columned text. 697pp. 8⅛ x 11. 22800-2, 22801-0 Pa., Two-vol. set $12.00

MECHANICK EXERCISES ON THE WHOLE ART OF PRINTING, Joseph Moxon. First complete book (1683-4) ever written about typography, a compendium of everything known about printing at the latter part of 17th century. Reprint of 2nd (1962) Oxford Univ. Press edition. 74 illustrations. Total of 550pp. 6⅛ x 9¼. 23617-X Pa. $7.95

PAPERMAKING, Dard Hunter. Definitive book on the subject by the foremost authority in the field. Chapters dealing with every aspect of history of craft in every part of the world. Over 320 illustrations. 2nd, revised and enlarged (1947) edition. 672pp. 5⅜ x 8½. 23619-6 Pa. $7.95

THE ART DECO STYLE, edited by Theodore Menten. Furniture, jewelry, metalwork, ceramics, fabrics, lighting fixtures, interior decors, exteriors, graphics from pure French sources. Best sampling around. Over 400 photographs. 183pp. 8⅜ x 11¼. 22824-X Pa. $6.00